Take Five!

How You Can Benefit from
Just Five Minutes
of Daily Exercise and
Start a Life-Long
Wellness Program

by
Sheila T. Cluff
Toni McBride
and
Mary Tabacchi

Take Five!

How You Can Benefit from Just Five Minutes of Daily
Exercise and Start a Life-Long Wellness Program

by Sheila T. Cluff, Toni McBride, and Mary Tabacchi.

160pp.

ISBN 0-9646248-1-8

Published by Fitness Two Publications, Ojai, CA

Edited, designed, and produced by Glenn Withiam

Printed in the United States of America by Elmira Quality
Printers, using vegetable-based ink on recycled paper with
at least 10-percent post-consumer fiber.

Acknowledgments

The authors would like to acknowledge the following contributions for their assistance with this project and book.

Cutter Cramton, Tammy Koehler, Dr. Margaret Jones, and Marjorie Sharpsteen—for their assistance with the Cornell University Study,

Guy Tabacchi—for his talents in producing the artwork

Debbie Gatch—for her secretarial support,

John Lauber—for his photographic assistance,

MaryAnn Stilwell—for her contributions to Chapter 1, and

The women and men from Cornell University who served as subjects for our study.

This book is dedicated to all the busy men and women in society who make a difference in this world and need a reminder from time to time to remember and value their own self worth; and especially to

Judy VanDermark,

who has given a new meaning to the words "purposeful living." Her vision, intelligence, and compassion make a difference as we hope this book will to all who read it.
—T.McB.

Foreword

In total, the authors have nearly 90 years' experience in the fitness and wellness fields. We have seen and heard just about every excuse for why exercise, or preparing more healthy meals, or reading a book for pleasure, or planting a garden is not possible in their lives at this time. Close to the top of the excuse list is **not enough time.**

Take Five! and the five-minute fitness program will help you eliminate this excuse from the list. We are pleased at the outcome of our study, and we want to pass on the good news regarding the beneficial effects of five minutes of exercise, self-esteem enhancement, and adherence to a lifelong habit of healthy practices that don't take a lifetime to be meaningful.

All of this is documented in the chapters of this book. Read on—and find out how you can improve not only your physical dimensions but the quality of your life. Our suggestions will add energy and strength, as well as mental, physical, and spiritual power to your life. The concept of wellness, as discussed in this book, is a lifestyle and a process. It's for everybody! And you can implement it at any time.

All that is necessary is your desire—and five minutes to start.

—Sheila Cluff, Toni McBride, and Mary Tabacchi

Contents

1. ❤

The Value of Activity

We have never met anyone who will argue that exercise is not good for you. Almost everyone will readily grant the value of exercise. But in the next breath, the excuses begin—excuses for why exercise is not in the picture for this person. Not enough time. No place to exercise nearby. Joint problems. Boredom with calisthenics or other repetitive exercises.

By one estimate no more than 20 percent of Americans actually exercise routinely three to five times per week for at least 30 minutes each time and achieve an appropriate heart-rate target. Forty percent are less active but do achieve health benefits from at least some exercise, and about 40 percent are presumed sedentary.[1]

We wrote this book because we found out that two of the most popular excuses for avoiding exercise—lack of time and potential boredom—don't need to be problems at all. You can get the full benefits of exercise with a program that takes you no more than five minutes each day. The only requirement of this program is that you exercise regularly.

We have all heard that to benefit from exercise you must "go aerobic" to achieve a physiological training effect. Aerobic exercise involves fairly vigorous movement for at least 30 minutes at a time. Running, bicycling, and swimming are typical aerobic exercises.

We don't have to tell you that today's lifestyle does not make it easy for most of us to maintain a schedule that includes a 30-minute daily run. Who really has the time to stop all other activity and go to a health club or other fitness facility to squeeze in the prescribed exercise session (plus a shower!) and then return to work? Most of us don't have that time. Moreover, if we try to cram all that activity into a one-hour lunch period (if we even have that long) exercise turns from entertainment to drudgery.

As we watched many of our associates struggle with their exercise programs, we started questioning the need for absolute adherence to the 30-minute aerobic guideline. We decided to test whether that was really only valid way for people to have the benefit of exercise.

The next chapter explains how we set up a study that demonstrated how just five minutes of activity can make a difference. Our test involved ordinary people—employees of Cornell University—who were not exercising at all before our study. As a result of that study, many of our test group kept right on exercising. Five minutes a day worked for them, and it can work for you.

Aerobic exercise promotes oxygen use in your body.

Sedentary lifestyle involves much sitting or inactivity.

Beyond Exercise

If all you do with this book is adopt our five-minute exercise routine, we will have accomplished what we set out to do, and you will benefit for the rest of your life. But we would like to encourage you to go beyond five minutes of exercise. In fact, we would like you to go beyond a simple focus on exercise to other aspects of a healthy lifestyle. This concept is called "wellness," and we will explain it throughout this book. So, if you are that busy person with barely enough time to breathe during your day, read on.

Most people realize that there is more to life than work. But then they'll say, "If you had my life, my spouse or partner, my children, or my boss, you would see how it's impossible to fit it all in." As we

Wellness is having a healthy, well-adjusted lifestyle.

work with people on wellness, we often hear such statements.

Consider this, though: no matter what your line of work might be, you will always have work to do. No matter how many hours you put in, there is always something more that can be done. You can count on the fact that the work will always be there!

That may not always be true of your health, however, especially if you let work dominate your life. Depending on the choices you make in your life your health might not keep up with your busy schedule. With the ideas in this book, we hope to help you stay as healthy as possible and delay the effects of aging.

Morbidity is another word for disease.

Balanced Fitness

None of us can avoid death, of course, but we can postpone what physicians call morbidity, which is the time of debilitating disease and painful decline that many people sadly experience. One of the ways to avoid or delay morbidity is with a healthy, balanced lifestyle that includes exercise. A noted expert, Dr. Steven Blair of the Institute for Aerobics Research, in Dallas, Texas, puts it this way: "If we start a balanced fitness program early in life, we'll be flexible enough to carry out our daily activities with no problems when we get older."

That is what we are talking about in this book— quality of life—or, how to blend all areas into the '90s way of living without compromising yourself during that quest for success. In fact, we urge you to define success much as Ralph Waldo Emerson did so eloquently in his essay entitled "Success":

> To laugh often and much; to win the respect of intelligent people and the affection of children; to earn the appreciation of honest critics and endure

the betrayal of false friends; to appreciate beauty; to find the best in others; to leave the world a bit better, whether by a healthy child, a garden patch, or a redeemed social condition; to know even one life has breathed easier because you have lived. This is to have succeeded.

Success by Emerson's measure starts from within. It does not include the usual items on life's score board, like titles, salary, and awards.

Fortunately, the literature on this topic shows that you can start working on this type of success any time. Regardless of when you put your body back into motion it will respond and improve both physiologically and psychologically.[2] Our bodies were designed to be in motion. Without activity the body decreases in size, becomes weak, and will fail. This is not new information for any of us. The key question is, how much activity is necessary to support our busy lifestyles?

The answer may surprise you. As little as five minutes of exercise performed every day is actually enough to affect us physiologically and, probably more important, psychologically. Before we give you our detailed discussion of the study we conducted, we would like to share the following story about an individual who served as a subject in our study and who best summarizes this point.

One Woman's Story

"I started in the research study two years ago at a weight of over 230 pounds, probably closer to 240 pounds. When you are that fat you never weigh yourself. This was the heaviest I have ever been and I carried most of it below my waist. I am 5' 5" tall and at that time in my life too busy to exercise routinely. I know people would stare and giggle as I walked by them. Once in New York City a man walked by me and called me 'very fat,' in Spanish. Since I understand Spanish I understood his insult. That really hurt.

"When I heard about the study and that I would only have to exercise five minutes a day, I signed up right away. I knew that something had to be done, and I thought that I would be in the company of other women who like me would be too embarrassed to be seen in shorts in a gym. The daily exercise in the privacy of my home helped me realize that with work I could improve my body and health. Every week I saw an improvement, however small that might be. It might be only one or two more repetitions, but to someone like me who had never done any exercising this was a big deal. I also noticed that I started to smile more and feel that maybe I could do something positive for my health and well-being. Then toward the end of the program I woke up one morning and I said to myself, 'You only have one body and you are the only one that can do something about it to make it stronger.' I know that for a lot of people this just makes sense, but for me it was the start of a new healthy lifestyle.

"After the study was completed I started going to the gym three nights a week and working out for only 20 or 30 minutes at a time. I would be exhausted. This was the first time in a long time that I had been in public, in shorts. Now, two years later I can fit entirely in just one leg of those same shorts. I joined a weight-management program and began to make modifications in my dietary practices. Today I can exercise aerobically for 1 to 1 1/2 hours and then lift weights. My attitude has greatly improved. I am not obsessed with food any more. Exercise has become a way of life. People who have not seen me in a year or so think that I look years younger. I even got my very first bicycle for my "thirty something" birthday. This spring I became unexpectedly ill and my doctor said that if I had not been in as good shape as I was I might not have survived my illness. This to me is all the proof I need to validate this lifestyle. Starting slow and regular was key to my success. Exercise was never important, necessary, or enjoyable. Today I would not live without it!"

Rethinking Exercise

Most people can relate to at least some part of this story. We found that many of the people in our study held similar attitudes about exercise, its role in their lives, and its importance. Most concluded that there just was not enough time to fit it all in. To the contrary, regular exercise seems to create more time. The more active and fit you become, the more you can accomplish in a fixed period of time. By learning to play as hard as you work, you can balance your "constant" workload with your personal life and set priorities for your lifestyle.

The value of activity on the human body is clearly understood. We wanted to test the effects of a certain level of activity. We hypothesized that exercise sessions need not be as long and vigorous as previously thought. Researchers have concluded that moderate exercise, activities requiring less than 60 percent of maximum aerobic capacity, offer many of the health effects as vigorous exercise.[3] Health-protective effects refer to such matters as improvements in heart function, reductions in blood pressure and resting heart rate, improvements in bone density, clearing of lymph system through muscle movement and sweating, and oxygenation of the blood system.

So it is that you can benefit from the common activities of daily living, such as walking and stair climbing, which have been shown to protect one from cardiovascular disease mortality[4] and to extend longevity.[5] Likewise, moderate exercise has also been shown to improve cardiovascular fitness. These moderate activities give most of the benefits of more vigorous activity but do not act as quickly as full aerobic workouts.[6]

The important point is, activity of any kind throughout a lifetime is key.[7] Statistics demonstrate that the majority of people will engage in many forms of moderate-intensity type activities throughout their lifetime. As people age they may engage in less vigorous exercise, but as long as they keep moving they will benefit.

That point returns us to our original notion that time constraints interfere with activity. People often cannot find the time even to walk the stairs (they take the elevator) or take a stroll to get lunch (they order in). That's why our five-minute program can be so important to you. It might be all you need to get started. And it's important for more than just your body. It also can help your mental state.

Mind-Body Connection

The relationship between exercise and our mental health has been recognized for many centuries. For example, Homer in ancient Greece declared, "*Mens sana in corpore sano*"—a sound mind in a sound body. Likewise, R. Burton observed back in 1632:[8]

> As too much and violent exercise offends on the one side, so doth an idle life on the other. . . Opposite to Exercise is Idleness or want of exercise, the bane of body and minde, . . the chiefe author of all mischiefe, one of the seven deadly sinnes, and a sole cause of Melancholy.

It has been reported by the American Psychiatric Association that 4.5–9.3 percent of females and 2.3–3.2 percent of males in the United States have a major depressive disorder. Depression has become one of the most common complaints of those who seek psychotherapy.[9] While it is beyond the scope of this book to delve into these findings, suffice it to say that today's version of success—so different from Emerson's—presents considerable pressures that often show up as depression.

Depression is low spirits or low vitality.

There has been much written today regarding the mind-body connection. What the mind possesses the body expresses. Addressing both physical as well as emotional and spiritual well-being is part of the big picture.

For a majority of this century much attention was given to the development of mood-altering drugs and the neurobiology of depression. We are beginning to see a shift back to the role of behavior in the prevention of disease and the promotion of health. This has refocused attention on the role of exercise in mental health.[10]

Many studies have supported the notion that exercise is associated with reduced depression.[11] The National Institute of Mental Health (NIMH) also has supported the positive influence exercise has on mental health. In 1987 a panel of experts with extensive research and clinical experience in exercise science and mental health was convened by the NIMH and made the following consensus statements:

- Physical fitness is positively associated with mental health and well-being;
- Exercise is associated with the reduction of stress emotions such as anxiety;
- Anxiety and depression are common symp-

toms of failure to cope with mental stress, and exercise has been associated with a decreased level of mild to moderate depression and anxiety;

- Appropriate exercise results in reductions in various stress indices such as neuromuscular tension, resting heart rate, and some stress hormones; and
- Current clinical opinion holds that exercise has beneficial emotional effects across all ages and in both sexes.

Although the exact effects of exercise on mental health are still debated by scientists today, our study seemed to support the notion that activity in general may improve an individual's mental outlook and self-esteem. As positive physiological changes occur an individual may be more likely to continue and progress through life with a healthy outlook and perspective toward what ever life has to offer.

Five Minutes...

As we said, the next chapter describes our study supporting the value of a five-minute exercise program. In following chapters, we show you how to progress if you decide to take the next steps: how to be "heart smart" and gain cardiovascular endurance, different modes of exercise to help you strengthen your muscles, and how nutrition fits into your exercise program. We'll also help you stay motivated to exercise and go into more detail on the concept of wellness, which will be part of your new definition of success.

...and Beyond

Life as we know it today is a tremendous challenge. But think of it this way: if you continue to do what you've always done, you'll always get what you've always gotten—and nothing will ever change for you. Our challenge to you is to try something different. Dare to be better! All activity has a positive effect on the mind and body. If you have no time and find exercise boring, read on, because it's easier than you think to make a change. You *are* worth it! ❤

References

[1] T. Stephens, D.R. Jacob, and C.C. White, "A Descriptive Epidemiology of Leisure-Time Physical Activity," *Public Health Reports,* 100 (1985), pp. 147–158.

[2] G.J. Pfeiffer, *Taking Care of Today and Tomorrow* (Reston, VA: Center for Corporate Health Promotion, 1989); and R. Rikkers, *Seniors on the Move* (Champaign, IL: Human Kinetics Publishers, 1986).

[3] J.F. Sallis et al., "Moderate-Intensity Physical Activity and Cardiovascular Risk Factors: The Stanford Five-City Project," *Preventive Medicine,* 15 (1986), pp. 561–568.

[4] R.S. Paffenbarger, A.L. Wing, and R.T. Hyde, "Physical Activity as an Index of Heart-Attack Risk," *American Journal of Epidemiology,* 108 (1978), pp. 161–175.

[5] R.S. Paffenbarger, A.L. Wing, R.T. Hyde, and C. Hsieh, "Physical Activity, All-Cause Mortality and Longevity of College Alumni," *New England Journal of Medicine,* 314 (1986), pp. 605–613.

6 W.L. Haskell, H.J. Montoye, and D. Orenstein, "Physical Activity and Exercise to Achieve Health-Related Physical-Fitness Components," *Public Health Report*, 100 (1985), pp. 202–212.

7 J.F. Sallis et al., "Physical-Activity Assessment Methodology in the Five-City Project," *American Journal of Epidemiology*, 121 (1985), pp. 91–106.

8 R. Burton, *The Anatomy of Melancholy* (Oxford: Ion Lidfield for Henry Cripps, 1632).

9 A.T. Beck, *The Diagnosis and Management of Depression* (Philadelphia: University of Pennsylvania Press, 1973).

10 U.S. Department of Health and Human Services, *Promoting Health/Preventing Disease: Year 2000 Objectives for the Nation* (Washington, DC: U.S. Government Printing Office, 1990).

11 See, for example: R.K. Dishman, "Medical Psychology in Exercise and Sport," *Medical Clinical North America,* 69 (1985), pp. 123–143; C.H. Folkins and W.E. Sime, "Physical Fitness Training and Mental Health," *American Psychology*, 36 (1981), pp. 373–389; W.P. Morgan, "Affective Benificence of Vigorous Physical Activity," *Medical Science Sports Exercise,* 17 (1985), pp. 94–100; C.P. Ransford, "A Role for Amines in the Antidepressent Effects of Exercise: A Review, *Medical Science Sports Exercise,* 14 (1982), pp. 1–10; and C.B. Taylor, J.F. Sallis, and R. Needle, "The Relation of Physical Activity and Exercise to Mental Health, *Public Health Report,* 100 (1985), pp. 195–202.

18 ❤ *Take Five!*

Glossary

Aerobic exercise—Exercise that promotes oxygen use in your body.

Calisthenics—Light exercises, usually repetitive, such as sit-ups and jumping jacks.

Cardiovascular system—Lungs, heart, and blood vessels.

Depression—Low spirits or low vitality.

Endurance—Capacity for prolonged activity.

Morbidity—Disease.

Neurobiology—The study of the nervous system.

Sedentary—Accustomed to sitting or inactivity.

Wellness—Having a healthy, well-adjusted lifestyle, with positive physical and mental frames of reference.

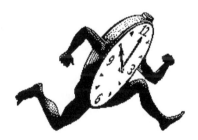

2.♥

The Five-Minute Fitness Plan

I f you are not currently exercising—or if you're not convinced that five minutes each day is enough to improve your fitness—the study in this chapter should convince you. And if you think you might like to start exercising but you just can't quite find the time, this chapter is especially for you. We'll explain the results of our study of people who weren't exercising but were interested in improving their wellness level (see chapter six for more about wellness). We believe that the results of the study apply both to people who exercise regularly and to those who have not had time to exercise. The exercises are particularly effective in strenthening abdominal and lower back muscles, all of which are so important in preventing back injuries and maintaining posture. As you will also see, there is a substantial psychological lift for people who stay with an exercise program like the five-minute fitness program.

To test our conviction that lengthy sessions of vigorous exercise were not the only way to gain the advantages of physical activity, we developed a small test study. We set out to determine how much exercise is necessary to elicit a physiological training effect on the human body and whether that effect would motivate an individual to continue exercising on the five-minute plan—or perhaps want to do even more. We designed the study to test two hypotheses relating to the physical and mental benefits of exercise. Our study involved asking people who were not exercisers to try the five-minute fitness plan.

The first hypothesis was that a daily routine of adhering to the five-minute fitness plan would improve three measurable physical-fitness factors: extensor flexibility, abdominal strength, and abdominal endurance. Those are three ways of assessing abdominal muscle tone, which is important in preventing low back pain and injury.

The second hypothesis was that the test subjects who stayed with the five-minute plan would experience improved psychological factors, such as self-esteem. A corollary of that hypothesis is that, as a result of the positive physiological and psychological changes, people would want to continue exercising.

We conducted our study among staff members at Cornell University in Ithaca, New York. Through the university's wellness program, we invited participation from employees between the ages of 21 and 55. To qualify for the study, a person had to be a non-exerciser for at least one year prior to the study and be living what the subject considered to be a sedentary lifestyle. The volunteers were then randomly assigned to either the experimental group or a control group. We started with 25 people in each group. Due to attrition, however, we finished the study with 13 people in the experimental group and 12 in the control group.

The study ran for 12 weeks. During that time, the subjects assigned to the experimental group were asked to perform the five-minute fitness plan each day. They were given a log card on which to record their exercising and were asked to mail it back in each week. The control group continued about their business and made no changes in their lifestyle.

Prior to the beginning of the 12 weeks all subjects took physical and psychological pre-tests, which served two purposes. The first purpose was to establish baseline physical-fitness and psychological measurements for both groups. Using those mea-

Hypotheses are assumptions or ideas to be tested.

Muscle tone is the condition of muscles. Good muscle tone implies firm muscles.

Self-esteem is a favorable opinion of oneself, but not at the expense of others.

surements, we could later determine whether the experimental group achieved any physical improvements and, if so, to compare those changes with the control group to see whether the changes were statistically significant. The second purpose was to be able to compare the groups of subjects to make sure that both groups had similar physical and psychological profiles at the beginning of the study. If one group were already more fit physically or psychologically, it would be difficult to draw any conclusions about the effectiveness of the five-minute exercise program.

Pre-Testing

Metabolism is the chemical processes in a person's body, particularly the use of energy.

For the physical-fitness test, we followed the well-established guidelines of the American College of Sports Medicine, a governing body for all exercise testing. We asked all subjects to follow a protocol consistent with those guidelines for three hours prior to testing. The protocol required that they not engage in any undue physical activity and that they not ingest any drugs (specifically, alcohol, nicotine, and caffeine) or food prior to the appointment. Eliminating the effect of these activities and substances on metabolism and heart rate would help rule out any major influences on the physical functions being tested.

We conducted the following tests:

- Resting heart rate;
- Resting blood pressure;
- Anthropometric measurements:
    —Height and weight,
    —Body-composition analysis (using skin-fold technique), and

Table 1

A Profile of the Test Subjects

	Experimental Group	Control Group
Number	13	12
Men	0	3
Women	13	9
Age Range	27–51	20–55
Mean Age	36	41
Pre-Test Comparisons		
Resting Heart Rate (beats per second)	76	73
Resting Blood Pressure (mmHg)	118/77	113/70
Weight (pounds)	162	159
Body Fat (percentage)	31	26
Waist Circumference (inches)	32	33
Hip Circumference (inches)	43	40
Flexibility (inches reached)	12	12
Sit-Ups (per minute)	27	29

—Circumference measurements (waist and hips);

• Modified sit and reach; and

• Modified curl up.

Table 1 shows the basic statistics for the two groups.

Tests Explained

We'll explain each test and the reason we applied it.

Resting heart rate is the number of times a person's heart beats in one minute in the absence of exercise or other provocation. Typical resting heart rates range from 60 to 100 beats per minute. We did not expect a subject's resting heart rate to change over the course of the study because our five-minute fitness plan is not cardiovascular exercise.

Resting blood pressure involves two readings that may be familiar to many people: systolic and diastolic pressure. Systolic blood pressure is the force against the artery walls when the heart contracts and pushes blood into the body. Diastolic blood pressure is the force exerted when the heart is between beats. Typical blood pressure readings are 100–120 mmHg (millimeters of mercury) for systolic pressure and 70–80 mmHg for diastolic pressure, commonly expressed as, for instance, "115 over 66."

Like resting heart rate, resting blood pressure is measured in the absence of exercise. While we also did not expect radical changes in blood pressure during the study, the American College of Sports Medicine guidelines required us to use the blood-pressure measurement as a screen for eligibility in the study. The guidelines set limits on which people may undergo testing or exercise programs on their own and who should not do so without medical clearance from a physician. Any subject found to have

Anthropometric measurements involve measuring the human body.

Body-composition analysis is an assessment of the relative amounts of lean and fat tissue.

high blood pressure or to be on the borderline was not permitted to participate in the study.

Anthropometric measurements are measurements taken on the size of the human body, such as height, weight, body-fat percentage, and circumference of the waist and hips. We measured body composition with the skinfold-caliper technique, in which various areas of a person's body are measured with a caliper by gently pulling the skin and fat tissue away from the muscle and putting the fold in the caliper. Through a series of calculations, the percentage of body fat can be estimated with a reasonable degree of accuracy. Once again, given the duration of our exercise program, body composition was not expected to change, but we could use the test to establish that both the experimental group and the control group were similar in physical measurements.

We took circumference measurements of each subject's waist and hips to see whether the five-minute fitness plan would create any differences between how the experimental group measured before and after the 12 weeks.

The final two tests were the *modified sit-and-reach* (SR) test and the *modified curl-up* test. These tests were chosen because they provide an indication of the health of a person's lower back and can indicate a person's susceptibility to experiencing back pain or injury. This is important because lower-back injury claims are America's number-one worker-compensation expense. For the most part, these claims are preventable, but the evolution of automation and technology is taking us in a direction of becoming more sedentary and less fit. Moreover, office equipment in the form of computer workstations can be

Skinfold-caliper technique is a means of assessing amounts of lean and fat tissue by gently squeezing and measuring a portion of skin and associated flesh.

The **sit-and-reach test** is a means of measuring flexibility by having a person stretch forward while sitting flat on the floor.

The **extensor mechanism** comprises the muscles that move arms or legs away from the body extremely hard on a person's lower back if the muscles that support the area are not maintained.

With a sedentary lifestyle, two physical parameters are compromised: extensor-mechanism flexibility, which involves the muscles that support our back from shoulder all the way to our Achilles' tendon, and abdominal strength. By sitting behind a desk or a steering wheel for most hours of a day your muscles begin to lose their compliancy, strength, and endurance. Contrary to what some people may think, such muscle loss is not the automatic effect of the aging process, but results mostly from a sedentary lifestyle.

As the muscles weaken, you can experience back pain without even injuring your back or leg. Just from sitting long hours you can over time begin to show symptoms and eventually rupture or herniate a disk from an otherwise benign movement. The good news is that just by getting active you can reverse this process and improve back health immediately.

A **flexometer** is a device for measuring muscle flexibility used in the sit-and-reach test.

The SR test is a common measure of back flexibility. A flexometer is used for this test. We asked each subject first to extend his or her arms fully forward with the legs extended straight, feet against the box, to set a mark for their reach. Then they were asked to slide the rule across the top of the box as far forward as they could go. The point at which they stopped or where their knees began to bend was the end mark. The difference between the reach and the end mark was their score. Using an initial reach negated the effects of shoulder mobility and limb-length bias so that all subjects could be accurately assessed for hip and trunk flexibility.

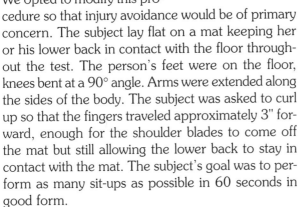

The 60-second modified sit-up test evaluated abdominal strength and endurance. We opted to modify this procedure so that injury avoidance would be of primary concern. The subject lay flat on a mat keeping her or his lower back in contact with the floor throughout the test. The person's feet were on the floor, knees bent at a 90° angle. Arms were extended along the sides of the body. The subject was asked to curl up so that the fingers traveled approximately 3" forward, enough for the shoulder blades to come off the mat but still allowing the lower back to stay in contact with the mat. The subject's goal was to perform as many sit-ups as possible in 60 seconds in good form.

Psychological Element

To test the psychological dimension, we administered a personality questionnaire called the Multidimensional Self Esteem Inventory (MSEI) to each subject. The MSEI was not meant to be a diagnostic instrument of any kind but rather to provide information regarding the personality traits of each individual as they relate to self sufficiency and body image. If a person's attitude improved as she or he experienced positive physiological changes, that person might be motivated to exercise more. For a complete definition of all components scored on the MSEI, see Table 2 (next page).

Table 2

The MSEI Self-Esteem Items

Each pair of items represents the extreme aspects of each category. Subjects taking the inventory indicated their "position" on each scale.

A. Global Self-Esteem

Pleased with self, feels significant as a person, self-confident, pleased with past, expects future successes.

Self-critical, dissatisfied with self, feels insignificant as a person, self-doubting, displeased with past, expects future failures unless major life changes are made.

B. Components of Self-Esteem

1. Competence

Competent, feels capable of mastering new tasks, learns quickly and does well at most things, feels effective and capable.

Incompetent, feels unable to master new tasks, learns slowly and often fails in difficult endeavors, ineffective, feels lacking in skills or talents.

2. Lovability

Worthy of love, feels cared for by loved ones, accepted as a person, can count on support from loved ones, able to express and receive feelings of love, involved in satisfying intimate relationship.

Unlovable, doubts that loved ones care, fears rejection because of certain personality aspects, unsure whether loved ones can be counted on for support, has difficulty expressing or receiving feelings of love, doubts about finding or maintaining an intimate relationship.

3. Likability

Likable, popular, accepted by peers and included in their plans, enjoyable companion, gets along well with others, popular in dating situations, expects to be liked, makes a good first impression.

Unlikable, unpopular, not accepted by peers and often excluded from peers' plans, has difficult enjoying being with and getting along with others, unsuccessful in dating situations, fears rejection, and often makes a poor first impression.

4. Personal Power

Powerful, successfully seeks positions of leadership, good at influencing others' opinions and behavior, assertive, has a strong impact on others.

Powerless, poor leader and avoids leadership positions, a follower who is strongly influenced by others' opinions and behavior, unassertive, rarely has a strong impact on others.

Adapted and reproduced by special permission of the publisher, Psychological Assessment Resources, Inc., 16204 North Florida Avenue, Lutz, FL 33549, from "Multidimensional Self-Esteem Inventory," by Seymour Epstein, Ph.D., and Edward O'Brien, Ph.D.

5. Self-Control

Self-disciplined, persevering, good at setting and achieving goals, not easily distracted, in control of emotions, exercises restraint in eating, drinking, and the use of drugs.

Lacks self-discipline, often fails to complete tasks, difficulty with setting and achieving goals, easily distracted, not in control of emotions, lacks self-control in eating, drinking, or the use of drugs.

6. Moral Self-Approval

Pleased with moral values and behavior, has clearly defined moral standards and acts in a way that is consistent with moral values, sets a positive moral example for others.

Guilty and displeased with moral values or behavior, unclear about moral beliefs and standards, often acts in an unethical or immoral manner, ashamed of setting a poor moral example for others.

7. Body Appearance

Physically attractive, pleased with appearance, feels that others are attracted because of appearance, feels sexually attractive, takes care to enhance physical appearance.

Physically unattractive, displeased with appearance, feels that others are repelled by looks, doubts sexual attractiveness, indifferent or unaware of ways to improve physical appearance.

8. Body Functioning

Well-coordinated, agile, in good physical condition, comfortable with body, enjoys physical activities such as dancing or sports, feels a sense of vitality and vigor in body functioning.

Awkward, clumsy, uncoordinated, in poor physical condition, uncomfortable with body, dislikes engaging in physical activities, feels unhealthy and that body is dull, lifeless, sluggish.

C. Identity Integration

Clear sense of identity, knows what he or she wants out of life, well-defined long-term goals, inner sense of cohesion and integration of different aspects of self-concept.

Confused, lacking a sense of identity and purpose, unsure of what he or she wants out of life, no long-term goals, much inner conflict among different aspects of self-concept.

D. Defensive Self-Enhancement

Defensive, overly inflated view of self-worth, claims to possess highly unlikely positive qualities, denies ubiquitous human weaknesses.

Open, non-defensive evaluation of self-worth, makes no claims of rare virtues, and acknowledges common human weaknesses.

With the testing over, we taught the five-minute fitness plan to those in the experimental group. Everyone had an opportunity to practice the technique with us so that they felt comfortable enough to do this at home on their own for the next 12 weeks.

Results

At the end of the 12-week study period, we reevaluated all 25 subjects with the same physical and psychological tests. We used statistical analysis to assess whether there were test-score differences between groups and within each group. Our analysis was conducted at a level of confidence that allowed us to be 95-percent certain that any differences we found were not due to chance.

In technical terms, we used t-tests to analyze our data. A p value equal to or less than .05 was used to establish statistical significance. The data on physical measurements are presented in Table 3 and the results of the psychological measurements are in Table 4.

The data provide strong evidence that the five-minute fitness test improved the experimental group's tests, particularly in extensor flexibility and abdominal endurance (Table 3). Mean values clearly illustrate the improvements the experimental (exercising) group experienced both physically and mentally. The before-and-after differences in extensor flexibility and abdominal endurance and strength among the experimental subjects were highly statistically significant. The p values at the .000 level tell us that these changes did not arise by chance. When compared to the non-exercising control group, the improvement in the experimental group's abdominal endurance is also statistically significant. Simply put, 12 weeks of exercise for just five minutes a day

Statistical significance is a mathematical calculation of certainty that a given study result did not occur merely by chance. Results are usually expressed as p values. A p less than .05 indicates no more than a 5-percent probability that a mathematical result occurred by chance.

Table 3

Changes During the Test

Experimental Group

	Pre-test	Post-Test	Sig. (p<)
Resting Heart Rate	76	78	.626
Resting Systolic Pressure	118	117	.938
Resting Diastolic Pressure	78	72	.018
Weight	162	162	.705
Percentage Body Fat	31	30	.495
Waist Circumference	32	32	.825
Hip Circumference	43	42	.001
Extensor Flexibility	**12**	**13**	**.000**
Abdominal Endurance	**27**	**47***	**.000**

Control Group

	Pre-test	Post-Test	Sig. (p<)
Resting Heart Rate	73	77	.331
Resting Systolic Pressure	113	116	.398
Resting Diastolic Pressure	70	71	.434
Weight	159	161	.008
Percentage Body Fat	26	26	.712
Waist Circumference	33	32	.190
Hip Circumference	39	38	.005
Extensor Flexibility	12	12	.189
Abdominal Endurance	**29**	**32***	**.054**

*Note: The difference between the two groups in post-test abdominal endurance is significant at $p < .01$.

Table 4

Psychological Trends (MSEI)

	Experimental Group		Control Group	
	Pre-Test	**Post-Test**	**Pre-Test**	**Post-Test**
Global Self Esteem	31	33	34	34
Competence	36	37	37	36
Lovability	36	36	36	36
Likability	35	36	36	37
Self Control	33	33	35	36
Personal Power	34	36	36	35
Moral Self Approval	41	44	44	42
Body Appearance	24	29	30	30
Body Functioning	24	29	30	31
Identity Integration	37	36	35	32
Defensive Self Enhancement	48	50	45	49

made a substantial difference for those who exercised, compared to those who didn't. The experimental group's improvement was consistent with our hypothesis that the five-minute fitness program can elicit physical improvements in the abdominal and lower-back muscles.

Members of the control group were actually less flexible after 12 more weeks of inactivity. T-test scores do not reflect direction, but only raw differences between the two groups. The post-test score differences between the two groups was not statistically significant, but the fact that the control group's flexibility score went down in the post-test is a strong testament to the real differences seen between the two groups at the end of the study.

As expected there were no differences of statistical significance within or between the groups on resting heart rate, resting blood pressure, weight, percentage body fat, or waist and hip circumference.

Mental Outlook

No significant differences on the groups' MSEI scores were found at the test's start. The absence of significantly different test scores on the pre-test allows us to conclude that the two groups were similar, and that the experimental group was no more motivated or in better psychological condition at the start than the control group.

The results of the MSEI further support the hypothesis that self-esteem may improve as physical-fitness characteristics improve. Of the 11 components of self-esteem that were evaluated using this test battery, the experimental group experienced statistically significant improvements in two areas: moral self-approval (p= .019) and body functioning (p = .018). These two attributes mean that a person is satisfied with her or his values and behavior and feels good about the body's physical functioning and condition. Such a person can be thought of as having a sense of vitality and vigor toward her or his body.

Note that a comparison of the trend demonstrated in the within-group analysis shows that only the experimental group experienced improvements in all 11 MSEI components, although the change was significant only in the two areas mentioned. The control-group analysis demonstrated no such findings and actually showed a decline in four areas (competence, personal power, moral self-approval, and identity integration).

The improvements in the experimental group's MSEI and the lack of improvement in the control group are important, because those findings support our hypothesis that the physical improvement from exercise improves one's attitude, and further can motivate a person to adhere to an exercise program. Probably one of the strongest pieces of evidence supporting that concept was that nearly half of the experimental group continued on with a fitness program after the 12-week study. Six months after the study, these people were still active. As an interesting note, all six who continued were women.

Speaking for Themselves

From a less scientific approach, the responses to the question asked of all subjects regarding how they felt about exercise is also strong support for our hypotheses. Remarkably all the subjects who began the study in both groups gave one of four answers: "exercise is boring"; "I do not have enough time"; "I do not like it"; or "I know it's good for me but ...."

The experimental group answered that question again following the study, with substantially different results. What most people came to realize was that time is indeed manageable. Here are a few samples of what some of our subjects had to say at the conclusion of the study:

- "I enjoy exercising when I can do it at my own convenience. This study has showed me that even a little exercise each day is really better than none at all."
- "I feel exercise is important only if it is constant and routine, not sporadic. I do believe if done regularly, the fear of lack of time goes away—good for self-discipline. Also, a routine is easier to develop than I originally thought when I started the program."
- "I don't really like doing it, but this exercise was fun and it wasn't time consuming."
- "I don't particularly like to do exercise, but when I am doing a routine of exercises at least three or four times a week I do feel more healthy. Basically I know it's good for me but I find it a chore."
- "I think everyone needs to exercise for good mental and physical health. The exercise program was very minimal and great for those who have been couch potatoes or have physical limitations."
- "I think exercise is a wonderful way to be good to oneself, and I feel good about myself when I do it."
- "I can do a limited program at my pace. I can enjoy exercise. I am glad I did this program as I gained self-esteem, gained bladder control, started a commitment and finished it, and participated in a project with helpful results.

It's good for me. I prefer to do it in private."

The five-minute fitness plan is an excellent routine for beginning an exercise program. It can elicit positive physiological changes and, in particular, improvements in extensor flexibility and abdominal strength and endurance—the very things that play key roles in preventing low-back pain or injury.

Probably the most exciting finding that came out of this study is the effect that even a small bout of exercise can have on the human psyche. When you feel better physically you usually feel better mentally. Even small amounts of exercise daily can instill a sense of accomplishment and self-approval.

Now, we are not claiming that five minutes of exercise will make your heart develop strength or help you burn many calories. This is purely a start. What we are suggesting is this: once you take that first step and begin to elicit physical and mental improvements, you will be ready for the next step... Being Heart Smart. ❤

References

American College of Sports Medicine, *Guidelines for Graded Exercise Testing and Exercise Prescription* (Philadelphia: Lea & Febiger, 1991).

D.D. Arnheim, *Modern Principles of Athletic Training* (St. Louis, MO: Times Mirror/Mosby College Publishing, 1988).

E.T. Howley and B.D. Franks, *Health/Fitness Instructor's Handbook,* Champaign (Illinois: Human Kinetics Publishers, 1986).

MSEI material adapted and reproduced by special permission of the publisher, Psychological Assessment Resources, Inc., 16204 North Florida Avenue, Lutz, FL 33549, from "Multidimensional Self-Esteem Inventory," by Seymour Epstein, Ph.D., and Edward O'Brien, Ph.D. Copyright © 1983, 1987, 1988 by Psychological Assessment Resources, Inc. Further reproduction is prohibited without permission from PAR, Inc.

Glossary

Achilles' tendon—A thick cord in the back of the ankle that controls much of the foot's movement.

Anthropometric measurements—Measuring the human body.

Body-composition analysis—An assessment of the relative amounts of lean and fat tissue.

Extensor mechanism—Muscles that move arms or legs away from the body.

Flexometer—A measuring device for muscle flexibility.

Hypotheses—Assumptions or ideas to be tested.

Metabolism—The chemical processes in a person's body, particularly the use of energy.

Muscle tone—Condition of muscles; good muscle tone implies firm muscles.

Self-esteem—A favorable opinion of oneself, but not at the expense of others.

Sit-and-reach test—A means of measuring flexibility by having a person stretch forward while sitting flat on the floor.

Skinfold-caliper technique—A means of assessing amounts of lean and fat tissue by gently squeezing and measuring a portion of skin and associated flesh.

Statistical significance—A mathematical calculation of certainty, usually expressed as a p value, that a given study result did not occur merely by chance. A p less than .05 indicates no more than a 5-percent probability that a mathematical result occurred by chance.

The Five-Minute Fitness Plan

...a quick, effective way to maintain flexibility and improve abdominal strength and endurance

General instructions: Perform each exercise for 30 seconds, unless otherwise instructed. Exhale throughout each movement.

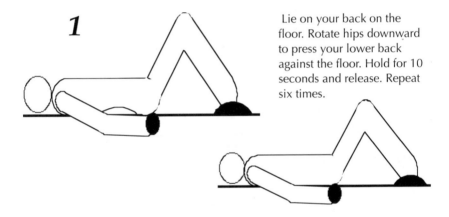

Lie on your back on the floor. Rotate hips downward to press your lower back against the floor. Hold for 10 seconds and release. Repeat six times.

Keeping your lower back in contact with the floor, arms extended forward on the floor, and knees bent, curl up until your fingertips travel about three inches forward from the start position.

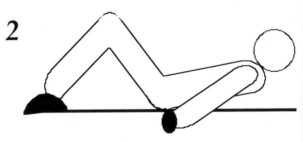

Keeping your back in contact with the floor, knees bent, one arm behind your head, and the other arm reaching straight out toward the opposite knee, curl up until your shoulder blades leave the floor for 15 seconds. Reverse arm positions and repeat for an additional 15 seconds.

3

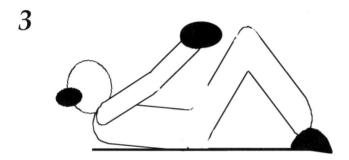

4 Keep lower back in contact with the floor. Starting with your right leg, push the right heel straight up and then bring your knee back to your chest, keeping your feet flexed. Alternate left and right, almost like a bicycle but using a straight, not circular motion. Gradually lower legs toward the floor, but do not lower past a 45° angle.

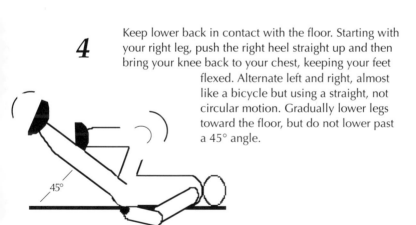

45°

Lying prone with each hand flat on the floor near your shoulders, press up until your elbows are straight. Your hips must stay in contact with the floor. Lower slowly back to the floor. The goal of this exercise is to extend your elbows all the way to build up the flexibility of your hip flexor, but when you are starting out extend your elbows only as much as your back and hips will allow.

5

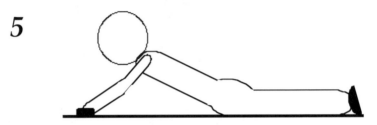

6

Sitting on the floor with your back straight, bend one leg but keep the other straight with your toe pointed up. Slowly bend forward from your hips, bringing your chest to your knee. Hold the position for 15 seconds on each leg. Remember to keep the stretching leg straight with your toe pointed up.

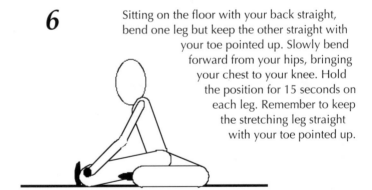

7

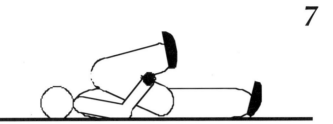

Lie flat on the floor with your head relaxed and knees bent. Grasp one leg behind the knee and pull toward your chest. Hold that position for 15 seconds. Switch legs and repeat for another 15 seconds. Remember to keep your head relaxed and on the floor.

8

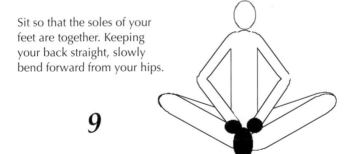

Still lying flat on the floor with your head relaxed and knees bent, grasp *both* legs behind the knee and pull toward your chest. Hold for 30 seconds, keeping your head relaxed.

Sit so that the soles of your feet are together. Keeping your back straight, slowly bend forward from your hips.

9

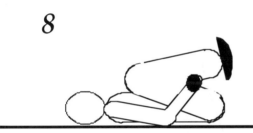

3.♥

The Next Step... Be Heart Smart

Congratulations! By moving on to this chapter, you have indicated your interest in taking the next step in building a health-oriented lifestyle. If you've been doing the five-minute workout regularly, you know how easy it is to make exercise a part of your life—once you get started.

While the five-minute fitness plan is valuable for improving your flexibility and abdominal strength, it is not designed to strengthen your cardiovascular system—your heart and lungs. The kind of exercise that strengthens your heart is aerobic activity, which is the next step in your progress toward total body fitness.

Aerobic capacity is the lungs' ability to take in oxygen combined the heart's ability to deliver the oxygen via the bloodstream to our body's cells. That oxygen is used to burn calories as our cells perform their functions. The product of this respiration process is energy. The more efficiently and effectively we metabolize our calories, the more energy we have to perform activities, be they physical or mental. This energy transfers directly into our activities of daily living (e.g., laundry, shopping, child care, lawn work, home maintenance) and to our responsibilities on the job (e.g., standing or sitting for long periods, paying attention in meetings, managing many tasks at one time).

Cardiovascular endurance is the proper term for your body's ability to continue producing energy and to perform your chosen activities with proficiency and without undue fatigue. Endurance is the base of physical fitness conditioning upon which other attributes, such as muscular strength and agility, are built. You can build endurance by exercising in a way that causes your heart and lungs to work harder than usual for a sustained period, usually 20 minutes or more. The particular mode of your aerobic activity (e.g., running, bicycling, swimming) is up to you and may depend on such other factors as the condition of your knees or the availability of a bicycle or swimming pool. As far as your heart and lungs are concerned, one exercise is basically as good as another, as long as a few training principles are followed. We will discuss those principles in a moment, but first, a word for readers who are not certain that they are ready for the next step.

Bicycling is an example of **aerobic exercise**.

We'll say more about these issues in our discussion of motivation (chapter five), but consider the following thoughts. The value of regular, moderate-intensity physical activity on the human body is well documented today. Exercise gives you substantial health benefits. It can help reduce stress, mitigate problems like high blood pressure, or cholesterol, and obesity, improve self-esteem and personal appearance, and, as we just mentioned, increase energy levels.

Obesity is a level of excess fat tissue that threatens health.

As we discussed in chapter two, we know it takes a personal commitment to get started. After all, we were once in your shoes and getting started with exercise. What we found—and what was experienced by the group in our study of the five-minute fitness program—is that the mental and physical benefits of exercise become a form of intrinsically driven motivation that keeps you going.

Intrinsic things are inside or within you.

In no time, you'll come to realize that you deserve this and you'll look forward to every activity session. Far from feeling like a chore, exercise will become part of your lifestyle. Nothing except an emergency will take its place in your schedule.

Many of us give so much time and effort to our families, friends, and colleagues that we have forgotten about ourselves. We say to ourselves: "When I have more time I will exercise and take more time to plan healthy meals." We would suggest that now is the time to make time.

For many of us, life's expectations have taken over. We try to be the successful business person, the perfect partner, the coolest and best Mom or Dad, the best housekeeper, the most savvy financial planner—and on and on. Many of us have allowed our inner being to get lost in the hustle and bustle of living in the '90s. It is time to reevaluate and take charge of our lives again.

Remember Emerson's definition of success. Take some time to put your health and well-being high on the priority list. As the advertising jingle used to say, "You deserve a break." And that break should come in the form of building your cardiovascular fitness. The more time and energy you put into feeling and looking more healthy and fit, the more mental and physical energy you acquire. Soon you realize you *can* have it all!

Now let's look at those training principles for aerobic exercise. We'll explore how much, how long, how often, and what kind.

How Much: *Intensity*

One of the ways of measuring how much exercise you are getting is by gauging its intensity. Intensity is the level of effort used to perform an activity. The intensity of aerobic exercise is measured by monitoring your heart rate in beats per minute. Different authorities suggest different percentages of your maximum heart rate as ideal for promoting improvements in physical and mental functions, a level known as your target heart rate, but those recommendations fall in similar ranges. The American College of Sports Medicine, for instance, recommends a heart-rate intensity of between 60 percent and 90 percent of your maximum heart rate.[1] The American Heart Association recommends 60 to 75 percent of maximum, while the Institute for Aerobic Research suggests a target heart rate of 65 to 80 percent of your maximum heart rate.[2]

We suggest that you exercise at an intensity that is comfortable and allows you still to talk to an exercise partner or trainer without being totally out of breath. This is called the "talk test." Somewhere in the range of 60–80 percent is usually acceptable.

The following formula will help you determine an appropriate target heart rate. It does not require you to guess what your maximum heart rate is.[3]

Karvonen's Formula for Target Heart Rate (THR)
THR = [(220 - age - resting heart rate) x training intensity] + resting heart rate

Here's how to use the formula:

A 44-year-old woman with a resting heart rate of 80 bpm is beginning an exercise program. She will start at an intensity of 60 percent (or .6). First she subtracts her age from 220 to get 176 (220 - 44 = 176). Then she further subtracts her resting heart rate of 80 bpm (176 - 80 = 96). Next she multiplies that number by her training intensity of 60 percent (96 x .6 = 57.6). Finally, she adds back her resting heart rate (57.6 + 80 = 137.6). Rounding this number, she finds that her target heart rate

Your **target heart rate** is a heartbeat pace that is appropriate or desirable during exercise.

at 60-percent intensity is 138 beat per minute. Repeating this formula and inserting .8 in the equation for an 80-percent training intensity, she gets a target rate of 157.

You probably won't want to stand there for an entire minute counting your pulse every time you check it. One further calculation makes it easier to monitor THR during your aerobic activity. Count your heart rate for ten seconds and multiply by 6. That gives you a quick, ten-second heart-rate check. Trying to count 138 or 157 beats over the course of one minute is unrealistic because your heart is beating fast. During exercise you can also count for 10 seconds and compare that number to your THR divided by 6. The woman in our example should be exercising between 23 and 26 for her ten-second count.

You can use any of several ways to monitor your heart rate. The safest and easiest method is to palpate your radial pulse along your wrist. To find this pulse place the end of the index and middle finger of one hand at the base of the thumb on your other hand right at your wrist joint. Slide your fingers towards the inside of your wrist until you feel a small groove between the first tendon of your index finger and the end of your wrist bone. Your radial artery lies right underneath this groove and you can count your pulse. Never use your thumb to count your pulse because your thumb and finger has a pulse of its own. Counting can be difficult if you feel two pulses.

Another method is to palpate your pulse at the carotid artery in your neck. Starting at your voice box slide your two finger tips away from the middle of your neck until once again you find yourself in a groove between the voice box and the first neck muscle (about an inch). Your carotid artery is the main blood supply to your brain, so press lightly to count pulses. Pressing too hard can actually slow the blood flow to the brain (a reflex in this artery in case of strangulation), which could cause you to feel light-headed or dizzy if you pressed long and hard enough.

Some people use electrical monitoring devices to monitor heart rate. These devices, ear lobe monitors or chest monitors, are available in most sporting-goods or exercise-equipment stores. Heart-rate monitors that use a strap around the chest and transmit the signal to a receiver around the wrist seem to offer the most accuracy. Consult your local exercise-equipment dealers for more information.

Don't be too concerned if you don't always exercise up to your THR. All activity is positive, as we have discussed. So all that happens if you don't exercise up to your minimum intensity is that you lose a little conditioning for heart strength.

A real concern arises, however, when you exercise out of your training zone, which presents issues of safety and health and fitness. Excess is not ideal when it comes to training the human body, so remember to monitor your heart rate to be certain that you are not exceeding your target heart rate. That will ensure not only a positive training effect but also a safe one.

To gain all the cardiovascular benefits we have talked about, your body needs to be using oxygen to burn calories and get energy to continue the activity. If your heart rate gets too high, your body begins to derive energy through other metabolic pathways and you no longer are in aerobic metabolism. Practically speaking, if you are in anaerobic exercise, as it's called, you do not burn fat calories as efficiently. Exercising in the recommended target heart rate ranges is the safest for your body and the best for burning fat.

How Long: *Duration*

Duration refers to how many minutes you exercise at your target heart rate. It is recommended to exercise continuously for at least 20 minutes (to achieve an aerobic effect). Longer is better for those with weight-management goals. Ideally a 45-minute aerobic exercise session is a good target, but remember that any amount of exercise is positive.

How Often: *Frequency*

Frequency refers to the number of times you exercise each week. The ACSM recommends a minimum frequency of three times per week of aerobic exercise, although five times per week is ideal. It is important for your body to have ample time to rest, recover, and rebuild its tissue between exercise sessions. That way, you get the full benefit of all the cardiovascular and mental-function improvements of exercise. The type of work your muscles experience during aerobic exercise is such that workouts can be performed on consecutive days as long as you take off one or two days during the week.

Once again, excess is not the goal. Extreme daily workouts are for Olympic athletes, not people like you who are going for lifelong conditioning.

What Kind: *The Exercise Session*

To ensure muscle efficiency and safety during exercise, follow this pattern during your workout.

1. *Warm-up.* To begin any workout session safely you should warm up. A warm-up is any activity that will prepare the body for your session with gradual increases in heart rate, blood pressure, and breathing rate. Warm-up activities should engage muscles that will be involved in your aerobic activity. For example, you might walk for five minutes before jogging or stair-stepping. A warm-up usually lasts from five to ten minutes. Your heart rate during warm-up should not be close to your target heart rate.

2. *Flexibility.* Flexibility exercise should be performed next to stretch out all major muscle groups in the body. Stretching may be the exercise procedure with the most misconceptions and misinformation. Adhere to the following tips when doing stretching exercises:

- Always hold stretches for at least 30 seconds and *do not* bounce to gain extra range of motion;
- Stretch slowly;
- Exhale as you lower into your stretches trying to think about the muscles being stretched and imagining them relaxing; and
- Systematically work down your body stretching the neck, shoulder, trunk, hips, back and legs.

The stretching routine illustrated on the next few pages provides a good pattern to follow.

The routine starts with neck stretches and then moves through the rest of the body.

Flexibility Exercises

...a stretching routine from head to toe

1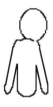

Neck: Slowly lower your head to each side and bring your chin to your chest. Caution! Avoid full neck circles and don't overextend your neck.

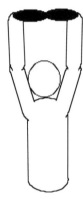

2

Shoulder and arm: Push your arms above your head and slightly backward, interlocking your fingers if possible. Always keep your back straight and your knees slightly bent.

3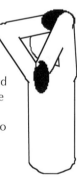

Triceps and shoulder: Bend elbow and reach behind and toward the opposite shoulder blade. Gently pull your elbow toward the opposite shoulder to enhance the stretching of your trunk. Once again, keep your back straight and your knees slightly bent.

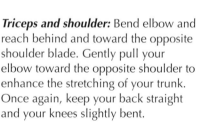

4

Upper back and shoulder:
With fingers interlaced, press your arms forward, opening the shoulder blades in the back. This time, keep your back slightly rounded and your knees slightly bent.

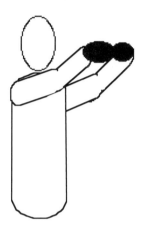

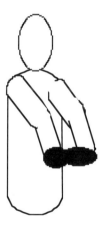

Chest and shoulder:
With your fingers interlaced behind your back, raise your arms as high as possible. Once again, keep your back straight and your knees slightly bent.

5

Lower back and buttocks: With your hands behind your knees and your head resting on the floor, pull your knees to your chest while keeping your lower back in contact with the floor.

6

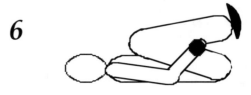

7

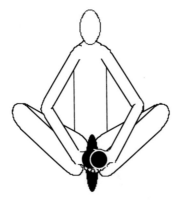

Inner thigh and groin: Place the soles of your feet together. Give gentle pressure with elbows to lower knees as you bend slowly forward from the hips. Keep your back straight!

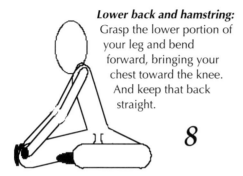

Lower back and hamstring: Grasp the lower portion of your leg and bend forward, bringing your chest toward the knee. And keep that back straight.

8

Quadriceps: Lying on your side, grasp your foot and pull toward your buttocks. To enhance this stretch, you can extend your entire leg back as you hold on to your foot. While keeping your back straight, rest your head on your arm, rather than propping it on your hand (hard on the wrist).

9

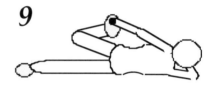

10

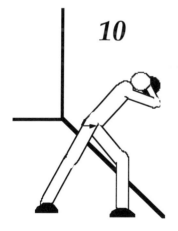

Calf and soleus: With feet flat and perpendicular to a wall, drive hips forward toward the wall. Stretch your rear leg in a straight position to stretch your calf (as illustrated) and then with your knee slightly bent to stretch your soleus. Your back should stay straight and your heels on the floor.

3. *Aerobic training session.* The key is to have fun! Pick activities that you really enjoy. Maybe it's something you used to do. Maybe it's something you've always wanted to try. The choice is yours; probably the more variety the better. Once again, the type of exercise is less important than monitoring your THR, maintaining appropriate duration, and exercising frequently enough each week for making sure you benefit from your exercise.

Walking is one of the best activities for beginning an exercise program. It is probably the most natural activity for most people and is the least likely to cause injury. Walking requires virtually no equipment outside of a supportive pair of exercise shoes. The shoes, incidentally, should be made with a comfort-cushioned inner sole and a shock-absorbent outer sole. Walking shoes are much stiffer than running shoes. You should consult your local sporting goods dealer for advice on shoes. In addition, various sporting magazines offer annual reports on top shoes including average prices. *Runner's World, Consumer Reports,* and *Shape* magazine are information sources. It is possible to get an adequate pair of shoes for around $40.

Walking is an excellent choice for persons with weight-management goals. Walking always burns calories, and if you walk long enough you can also burn stored fat. Here's an example. If a 170-pound person walks for 30 minutes, three times per week, in about seven weeks he or she will burn off one pound. If that person added one additional session per week, she or he could lose ten pounds in a year of walking.[4]

Different activities, of course, burn different calorie amounts. Taking the case of a 190-pound person, for instance, here is the length of time that person would have to perform various activities to burn enough calories to lose a pound. She or he would have to clean for just over 12 hours or take a leisurely bike ride for just under 12 hours. That pound would disappear after just under 7 hours of tennis, 6 hours and 45 minutes of pushing a lawnmower, and 6 hours and 30 minutes on a Universal gym. If you're a little lighter, you'll burn fewer calories for every minute of exercise, while a heavier person will burn a few more calories.

If you decided to give walking or jogging a try, it is almost inevitable that you will be traveling streets and highways. Keep these safety tips in mind:

- Always carry a quarter with you to be able to make a phone call if necessary.
- Vary your walking or jogging routes not only for personal safety, but also for variety and to minimize physical injury that might occur due to banked roads or uneven surfaces.
- Do not run in the evening if possible. Wear reflective clothing and shoes if you will be running in the evening.
- Walk or run with a partner or at least let friends know where you will be going and when to expect your return.
- Wear appropriate clothing for the weather conditions:
  —Light-colored, breathable material during hot, humid weather.
  —Layers of clothes during colder weather so that you can take off clothes as necessary to minimize chilling.
  —Rain-repellent or windbreaker clothing during inclement weather.

- Avoid "Walkman" headsets for two reasons:
  - —They can block out sound, which could put you in danger if you cannot hear warning sounds.
  - —The noise pollution developed from prolonged listening with headsets may produce irreparable damage to your inner ear.
- Walk and run against (facing) traffic.
- Carry identification.
- Drink plenty of fluids (water is best) before, during, and after exercise. Consider the temperature and the humidity level and hydrate appropriately. Thirst is not a good indicator of your body's hydration level. When you are thirsty, you are almost always beginning to dehydrate during exercise.

Once again, whatever your choice of mode of activity might be, remember to make it fun!

4. *Cool down.* The final part to your workout should be the cool down. Don't leave this part out! It is extremely important to slow down gradually after exercising and stressing the cardiovascular system. When you exercise, your muscular system assists your cardiovascular system in delivering the fresh, oxygenated blood to the body cells that need it and in returning the deoxygenated blood back to the heart to be pumped back up to the lungs and repeat the circulation process. When you stop exercising abruptly, your muscles stop assisting the heart. You can place undue strain on the heart by requiring it to pressure the whole system and keep blood moving at the speed and volume necessary for recovery. Staying upright and moving around is all that is required for ample cool down. As an example, after briskly walking in your target range, you could cool down with a casual stroll until your heart rate is at least in the low 100s. Whatever your choice of activity, slowly walking afterwards or performing the same activity slowly is key. Cool down at least three to five minutes or until your heart rate drops to the low 100s.

Progression Guidelines

This is another fun part to your programming ideas. Don't feel that once you choose an activity that's all you'll ever do for your exercise program. Experiment with many activities. If you work with exercise machines, vary speed, duration, and level. Change scenery and terrain when exercising outdoors. The sky is the limit to what you can do. Remember it's the target heart rate that dictates intensity.

Increase duration slowly. It might be a good idea to add one minute to your session every time you work out until you reach your target goal of 30–45 minutes. If weight management is also a goal, adding another exercise session to your weekly workouts is also an option.

Always remain in the zone of your target heart rate. As your body begins to become more conditioned, you will begin to notice that it requires more work to elevate your heart rate. At this point, it is not necessary to continue adding duration or frequency to your program in order to improve. That improvement will come as a result of increasing your intensity to achieve your THR. It's a good thing, too! Otherwise, a regular exerciser would have to continue adding time to sessions to improve cardiovascular endurance. Before long a person would have to be exercising many hours to get improvement.

The only reason to increase your duration would be if the goals of your program are stress reduction or weight loss.

Travel Fitness Kit

One final note on exercise for people who travel frequently and are not convinced a regular exercise program is possible. How about a travel kit for fitness-on-the-go that you take with you regardless of where you are going? With such a kit you could continue your program no matter how much you have to travel, but you will not have to rely on the presence of a fitness facility at your destination. You will also always have the equipment that is right for you.

Choose a bag for your exercise kit that will travel easily with you, will protect its contents if checked through an airport, is waterproof, and can be secured if you will not be able to keep it with you during the trip. We would suggest the following items for your travel exercise kit:

1. Exercise clothing that is appropriate for your destination.
2. Proper footwear for your chosen activities. If you will be walking or jogging, inquire from the hotel staff regarding safe routes around the area. Never venture out alone after dark regardless of how well lit the paths might be.
3. If you know of facilities available where you are staying, bring the appropriate exercise equipment (e.g., racquetball racket, golf clubs).
4. Take a tape player and extra batteries for warm-up periods. Include a variety of tapes regarding fitness, stretching, walking, and motivation. Don't forget some relaxation or inspirational tapes for unwinding following those busy days on the road.

5. If you know that a VCR will be available, include some exercise videos that you could do in the privacy and safety of your own room.

6. As part of any good cool down, don't forget the bubble bath or body splash to revitalize!

Whether you are at home or on the road, explore new activities. Exercise can be enjoyable yet make you work at the same time. Think in terms of lifetime exercise and put as much variety into your program as you feel comfortable with. Have you ever hiked a mountain? Have you ever ridden a mountain bike through the woods? Have you ever ridden a horse along the surf on a beach? Have you ever considered joining your community's summer softball, volleyball, or basketball league? Have you given in-line skates a shot? Would you consider planting and maintaining a garden for the next growing season? All of these activities can be a part of your exercise program. We challenge you to tap into your creative side and explore!

When you've made aerobic exercise a part of your lifestyle, you may be ready to expand your program again. How about the next step—weight training? In chapter four, we want to pump you up! ❤

References

[1] American College of Sports Medicine, "Position Statement: The Recommended Quantity and Quality of Exercise for Developing and Maintaining Fitness in Healthy Adults," *Medicine and Science in Sports*, 22, No. 2 (April 1990), pp. 265–274.

[2] K.H. Cooper, *Running without Fear: The Comprehensive New Guide to Safe Aerobic Exercise—Running, Swimming, Cycling, Skiing, and More* (New York: Bantam, 1985), p. 104.

[3] Vivian Heyward, *Advanced Fitness Assessment and Exercise Prescription* (Champaign, IL: Human Kinetics Books, 1991), pp. 79–81.

[4] Based on data from: E.W. Bannister and S.R. Brown, "The Relative Energy Requirements of Physical Activity," in *Exercise Psychology*, ed. H.B. Falls (New York: Academic Press, 1968); and R. Passmore and J.V.G.A. Durnin, "Human Energy Expenditure," *Psychological Reviews*, 35 (1955), p. 801.

Glossary

Anaerobic exercise—Physical exertion that does not promote the use of oxygen by the body, usually characterized by short bursts of activity.

Carotid artery—The vessel that supplies blood to the head and is easily found in the neck to count pulse rate.

Dehydration—Loss of water in the body.

Duration—The length of time exercising at the target heart rate.

Frequency—The number of exercise set in a week.

Hydration—Volume of water in the body.

Intensity—The level of effort used to perform an activity.

Intrinsic—Inside or within.

Obesity—A level of excess fat tissue that threatens health.

Radial artery—The vessel that supplies blood to the hand and is easily found in the wrist to count pulse rate.

Respiration—The use of oxygen by body cells to create energy.

Target heart rate—A heartbeat pace that is appropriate or desirable during exercise.

4.

Pumping Up

Muscular strength and endurance is another physical fitness measure that you might consider when looking at total body health. Muscular strength is defined as a muscle's ability to exert maximum force in a single all-out effort or in a few repetitions. Strength is important in maintaining the lean tissue of the body—bones, muscles, organs, and other soft tissue—because it helps maintain muscle tone and also helps promote bone density and strength of ligaments and tendons.

A chief reason to maintain lean tissue is its role in regulating your metabolism. The more lean tissue you have, the higher your metabolic rate and the more calories burned. Assuming an individual maintains healthy dietary practices and activity levels, a faster metabolism means that weight is easier to maintain. If your goal is to lose weight, a faster metabolism means faster weight loss. The more you work out, the more lean tissue (muscles) you will have and the faster your metabolism.

Strength training is a wonderful adjunct to your aerobic exercise program that helps strengthen not only your muscles but also bones, ligaments, and tendons—all of which get a workout when you're involved in aerobic exercise. Retention of lean tissue as one ages—and avoiding fat—is also beneficial to maintaining the activities of daily living and just plain feeling good.

Keep in mind that strength training does not necessarily mean building large muscles. In fact, women cannot build large muscles due to their lack of large amounts of testosterone. That does not mean, however, that a woman cannot have more well-formed or sculptured muscles.

Metabolism is the chemical processes in a person's cells that generate energy.

Strength training is becoming popular in nursing-home recreational programs and at senior centers. Your muscles can become stronger and more efficient at any age. Many geriatric studies have shown that increases in muscle mass are possible at any age. Moreover, people with stronger muscles were more capable of performing the activities of daily living and had a better mental outlook.

Pick the type of **strength training** that suits you best.

There are many different modes of strength training. Before deciding which type would best suit you, you should first understand the three methods of strength training—isometric, isotonic, and isokinetic.

Isometric training, or static lifting, involves contracting your muscles against an immovable object. Examples of isometric exercise would be pressing the palms of your hands together as hard as you could to strengthen the muscles across your chest, or pushing against a wall. This type of exercise promotes increases in muscle size, but strength gains are made only at the angle at which the joint works. This technique is useful in a rehabilitation setting where, for example, your leg might be in a cast or immobilizer. It helps slow down the atrophy (shrinking) that occurs in muscles when you cannot use them. From a practical standpoint, the value of isometric training is limited, since it enhances the muscle in a single direction while most activity occurs around movement of joints throughout many ranges of motion.

Testosterone is a male hormone that among other things causes muscles to develop.

Isotonic training or dynamic lifting has a much wider application than isometric training. Isotonic training involves contracting and lengthening a muscle throughout a range of motion while moving a load. While the load is constant in this kind of training, the force applied by the muscle varies as it moves through the range of motion. This is the classic form of weight lifting. An example is a biceps curl, or holding a weight in your hand, bending your elbow fully to lift it and then lowering it again (see page 75). This is a practical method of training your muscles because you gain strength around the range of motion.

Isotonic lifting often involves weight-lifting equipment or machines. Many types of equipment are available for this form of training, including machines (e.g., Universal, Nautilus, Keiser & Eagle, Gravitron), free-weight equipment (e.g., dumbbells and weight bars), and resistive exercise tubes. The type of equipment you choose for this exercise is a matter of personal preference.

Ligaments bind bone to bone, while tendons connect bones with muscles.

Exercise machines offer one feature that is not available from free weights or exercise tubes. Machines are designed to take the major pressure away from the joint and allow the muscles through a cam, pulley, or hydraulic system to exercise the joint as evenly as possible throughout the range of motion. Your muscles do not need to balance the weight because the machine does that for you. For this reason, machine lifting is less risky than the other two forms of isotonic exercise.

Free weights and exercise tubes have an advantage over machines, however, because they strengthen tendons and ligaments. Weights and tubes involve lifting the weight while balancing the load. Proper technique is critical to preventing injury, since you have control of the load. Tendons, ligaments, and the joint capsule (the tissue surrounding a joint) are strengthened while the muscle works. The choice of one isotonic method over another depends on the goals of your lifting program. An individual interested in strengthening not only muscles but joints and soft tissue should pick free weights and tubes or bands over machinery.

Isokinetic lifting can be performed only on specialized equipment usually found in a clinical setting such as a physical-therapy office. Isokinetic exercise controls speed of movement and provides accommodating resistance throughout the full range of motion, allowing the muscles to exert full or constant force. This type of training is effective in rehabilitating injured joints or training for a specific speed of movement in an athletic endeavor. An example of this equipment is Orthotrons or Cybex machines. Because of the specificity of the work performed in these machines they are expensive and typically found only in a clinical setting.

In part, the method of lifting you choose depends on the results you are looking for. Most people using strength training are seeking improved strength, toning, or power. You can achieve all three of these, but different types of lifting are required for different results.

Strength means developing your muscles' ability to lift maximum weight in a single all out effort or over a few repetitions. Usually a muscle's size or circumference increases as strength improves.

Power involves explosive action of the muscles or their ability to exert force with speed. Examples of this are your ability to swing an axe forcefully and repeatedly to split wood or a basketball player's ability to rebound with conviction.

Toning, or muscular endurance, is your muscle's ability to contract repeatedly against a light to moderate load. This type of exercise helps firm muscle tissue and allows you to be more efficient in activities of daily living such as carrying groceries, doing yard work, walking, or being on your feet for long periods of time. This type of training can also assist many types of aerobic activity.

When you have chosen the type and goals of training, your workout can be designed for optimal benefits. The design of the workout will specify volume, intensity, and frequency.

Volume is the amount of training you do, as measured by the number of repetitions and sets of repetitions completed on your particular weight-training equipment. A repetition is defined as a single complete action of an exercise from the starting point through the lift and back to the starting position. For example one repetition of a straight leg raise is to start with your leg on the ground and your body lying flat, lift the leg up to about a 45-degree angle, and return it to the ground. A set is defined as a given number of consecutive repetitions. An example is to do ten straight leg raises in a row for one set. It is usually written like this: 1x10.

Intensity is how much weight you lift in a given exercise. For strength you generally lift heavy weights, while power conditioning requires moderate weight, and lifting for muscular endurance requires lighter loads. The correct amount of weight is difficult to determine in advance, although trainers and books can give you recommendations. Once you have decided on the number of sets and repetitions in a set, you should choose a weight that will fatigue your muscles as you complete the set. For example, if you were trying to build strength in your biceps muscle (with a volume based on the recommendations in Table 1, page 69), you would choose a weight that you could not lift any more without breaking proper form as you approach repetitions six through eight. You should always exercise a muscle to fatigue rather than stop at the predetermined number of repetitions in that particular set.

Always take a rest interval between sets. This period varies according to the type of exercise you have chosen. Weight training has different effects on your muscles than aerobic training and a different recovery period from one workout to the next. Although you can easily handle a frequency of up to five times a week in consecutive sessions with aerobic training, weight training requires a different level of recovery. We recommend lifting no more than three times per week with at least one day of rest between workouts. Table 1 illustrates the recommended variables for each of the three types of weight training.

Regardless of the method and type of exercise, weight training activities should be performed in a particular order. A well-rounded program includes at least one exercise for each major muscle group of your body. You should arrange your exercises so that muscle groups have time to recover as you move along through your program. Lifting from largest muscle groups to smallest is also recommended. Remember always to exercise opposing muscle groups equally. Opposing muscles work together and should stay in balance to reduce risk of injuries. We have

Deltoids
Trapezius
.Rhomboids
Triceps
Spinal erectors
Latissimus dorsi
Tensor fascia latae
Gluteus maximus and medius ("gluts")
Hamstrings
Gastrocnemius
Soleus

Posterior view of human muscles

already discussed the contribution of weak abdominal muscles to lower back pain. Both the lower back muscles and abdominals are important in keeping the spine in alignment and keeping the disks between vertebrae in proper position.

Examples of opposing muscle groups are the following:

- biceps–triceps,
- deltoids–latissimus dorsi,
- pectorals–rhomboids and trapezius,
- quadriceps–hamstrings, and
- abdominals–spinal extensors

Progress through your workouts slowly, and never sacrifice form for more weight. To make progress in your program change only one variable at a time: load, repetitions, or sets. We recommend increasing reps or sets before adding more load. When you increase load expect to decrease the number of reps that can be performed per set at the onset. Again as muscular strength or endurance develop you will once again perform the same amount of sets and reps and progress up again. Remember recovery time between sets and the order of lifting are both important. Alternating between upper and lower body and from larger to smaller muscle groups is ideal. Table 2 (page 73) gives an example of this pattern.

Regardless of the type of equipment you use, we urge you to adhere to the following training principles, not only for your safety but to ensure an efficient workout session.

- Always warm up. Prior to lifting, warm up your entire body and the muscle groups that will be worked. Five to ten minutes is usually appropriate. As with aerobic activity, stretch out after

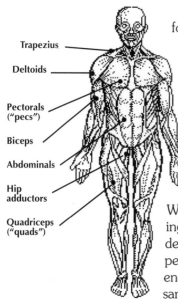

Trapezius

Deltoids

Pectorals ("pecs")

Biceps

Abdominals

Hip adductors

Quadriceps ("quads")

Anterior view of human muscles

warming up. If you are doing a cardiovascular workout on the same day as weight training, do the aerobics first.

- Lift the resistance or weight faster than you return it, but do everything in a controlled manner with perfect form. A recommended rate is lift in two counts and return in four counts.
- Work smoothly and throughout the full range of motion. Do not lock out, or fully straighten knees or elbows when lifting with these joints.
- Always exhale while lifting the resistance and inhale at the start of a lift or through the return phase.
- As you exercise, think about the muscles you are using and feel them moving and exerting force. Concentrating on form and muscle movement is another type of mental training and is a valuable tool to develop along with the muscle strength or endurance.

Table 1

Strength-Training Program Design

Goal	Repetitions	Sets	Rest Interval	Weight*
Strength	3–8	1–3	2–4 minutes	Heavy
Power	6–10	1–3	1.5–2 minutes	Moderate
Endurance	10–15	1–5	45–90 seconds	Light

*Note: The load varies with the type of program you wish to follow. A heavy load, used for strength training, is one you can lift three to eight times in a set and no more. Moderate resistance, used for power training, is a weight for which the last two or three of the ten repetitions is difficult. A light weight, used for endurance training, is one that can be lifted repeatedly with little difficulty.

- If you experience pain while lifting, reduce the resistance (intensity) and reevaluate your form. If pain persists, stop the exercise and consult your physician. A mild burning sensation is expected but should subside as the exercise is finished. Soreness the next day is fairly common with beginner programs. An additional day or two of recovery time may be necessary. Listen to your body.
- Proper nutrition and sleep is critical for any exercise program and, indeed, for proper functioning in all activities.
- We strongly recommend that you keep records of your exercise. Track the type of exercise, number of sets and repetitions, date of workout, and amount of resistance used (if known). Add comments—jot down your feelings and observations from time to time. Record keeping is an excellent motivational tool as well. See Table 2 for an example.

Muscles develop strength and endurance from overload. To improve your muscles, you must stress them over their normal limits without damaging them. As you progress through your program you will continually need to make adjustments in your resistance to accommodate your improvements. This concept, known as progressive resistance, is similar to increasing the intensity of aerobic exercises. Record keeping is helpful in gauging your progress. You can refer back to your notes and make adjustments in your program systematically based on actual results.

Muscles also respond when they are exercised in a particular manner, termed specificity. If you want to gain strength in the upper body, all the major muscles should be included in your program: chest, shoulders, arms, back, and neck. As you plan your program consider not only the type of equipment, volume, and intensity but also overload, progressive resistance, and specificity.

Now you are ready to begin. We have included a sample program on the next few pages using elastic tubing as your mode of exercise. This "equipment" is virtually free if you have an old bicycle tube lying around that you can cut in half and use. If not, visit your local bicycle repair shop. Most are more than willing to give you a punctured tube. Exercise tubes are also commercially available in most sporting goods stores and are usually sold with varying resistive loads (light, medium, or heavy).

We also present a sample weight training program. If you are beginning a training program, light or medium resistance is appropriate. The following program would make an excellent adjunct to your cardiovascular program or to your five-minute exercise session. Remember to breathe, maintain technique, direct your thoughts—and enjoy moving your body. That enjoyment is a big factor in maintaining motivation, as we'll discuss in the next chapter. ❤

Glossary

Geriatric research—Studies of aged people.

Isometric training—Exercises involving pushing against or pulling unmoving objects.

Isotonic training—Exercises involving lifting a load to move a muscle through its full range of motion.

Isokinetic lifting—Exercises that move muscles in specific ways using specialized equipment.

Ligament—Connective tissue that joins bones in joints.

Muscle tone—The muscle's ability to contract repeatedly against a moderate load.

Opposing muscles—Muscles working in pairs opposite each other. Usually one extends and the other retracts.

Repetitions—Repeated controlled movements to exercise a particular muscle or group of muscles.

Range of motion—The distance within the limits of a muscle's ability to move.

Weight Training Log Card

Write: Sets/Replications

Session				
1. Bench press (pectorals)				
2. Leg press (combo lower body)				
3. Shoulder press (deltoid/triceps)				
4. Leg extension (quadriceps)				
5. Lat pulldown (latissimus dorsi)				
6. Leg curl (hamstrings)				
7. Seated rowing (latissimus dorsi, biceps)				
8. Shoulder shrug (trapezius, rhomboids)				
9. Calf raises (gastrocnemius and soleus)				
10. Upright rowing (deltoids, trapezius, biceps)				
11. Triceps extension (triceps, latissimus dorsi)				
12. Lateral raises (deltoids, trapezius)				
13. Crunches/Sit-ups (abdominals)				

Tube exercises	Session			
1. Horizontal arm pull				
2. Biceps curl				
3. Triceps extension				
4. External rotation of shoulder				

Sample Tube Exercises

The following are examples of exercises that can be performed with exercise tubes. Remember to execute these safely and use good form. Keep your back straight, knees slightly bent, feet shoulder width apart, chest forward, and shoulders even. Make sure to control the return movement.

Experiment with your tube and be creative. You can exercise almost all your muscle groups this way. Start by exercising large muscle groups first and then the smaller ones, making sure to alternate groups.

Horizontal arm pull

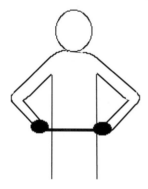

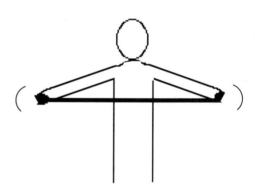

With arms in front of body, start by pulling with minimal tension on the band.

To finish, extend arms laterally to an open chest position and then ease back to starting position.

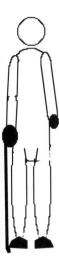

Biceps curl

Start with tension on the band and your elbow slightly bent (as at left). Stand on one end of the band and pull the other end up even with your shoulder (right), bending the elbow and keeping it tight by your side. Then repeat with your other arm (below).

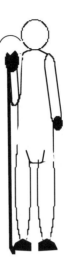

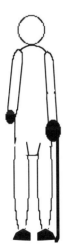

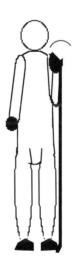

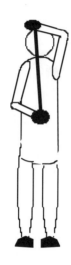

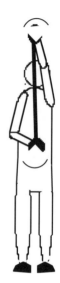

Triceps extension

Working behind your back, start with your left hand holding one end of the tube and your right hand behind your head holding the other end. Raise your right arm straight over your head, extending the tube.

After gradually allowing the tube to contract, change hands and repeat, extending your left hand over your head.

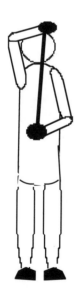

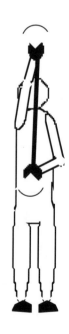

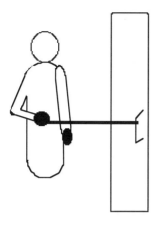

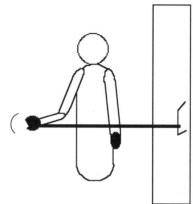

External rotation of shoulder

Tie one end of the tube to a door knob. Keep your elbow close to your body and bent at 90°. Using that hand, hang on to the tube with a slight tension. Keeping your elbow close to your body, rotate the arm out so that your shoulder joint rotates externally. Face the opposite direction, change hands, and repeat by rotating opposite shoulder.

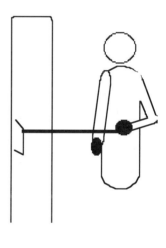

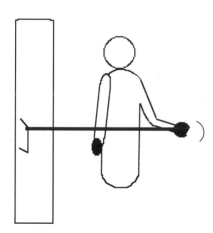

A Sample Weight-Training Program

These lifts exercise each major muscle group in an appropriate order. Generally, unless otherwise instructed, keep your back straight and your elbows and knees flexed. The number of sets and repetitions depend on the goals of your program. Table 2 will help you set up a program.

Bench or chest press (pectorals)

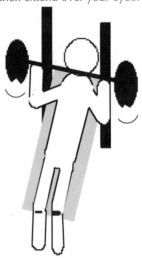

Keep your feet flat on the floor and your shoulder blades and hips in contact with the bench. Hands are positioned shoulder width apart on the bar. Lower bar toward chest and then extend over your eyebrows.

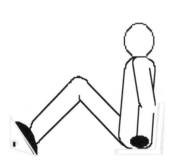

Leg Press (quadriceps, hamstrings, gluteals)

Using a Universal or similar machine, put the balls of your feet on the platform and hips against the seat. Extend your your legs forward keeping at least a slight bend in the knee. Return to the start position with control.

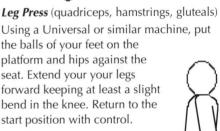

Shoulder press (upper back, neck, triceps)

Start with bar resting behind neck and arms wider than shoulder width, supporting the weight off the back of the neck. Extend your arms up over your head, controlling the bar. Return to start with control.

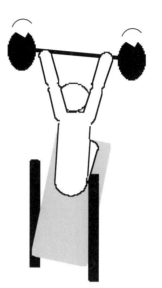

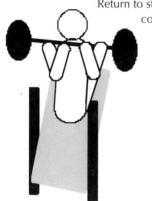

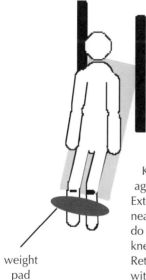

Leg extension (quadriceps)

On a Universal machine, start with knees bent at a 90° angle and weight pad comfortably placed above your feet so that it doesn't limit your legs' extension. Keep back straight against support pad. Extend legs forward nearly to level, but do not lock your knees completely. Return to start with control.

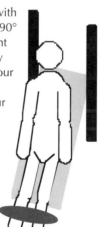

weight pad

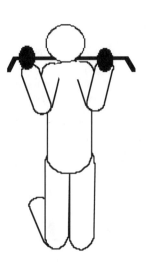

Latissumus pulldowns (latissimus dorsi)

Using a Universal or free-weight machine, grasp the bar with arms extended at shoulder width. Pull down behind neck approximately to shoulders. This move is usually performed while kneeling or sitting.

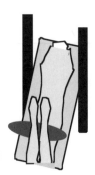

Leg curl (hamstrings)

On a Universal or free-weight machine, lie on your stomach, placing your legs under the weight pad just above your Achilles tendon. Keep your knees slightly bent. Curl both legs to a 90° angle, keeping hips and chest in contact with pad. Control the return to the start position.

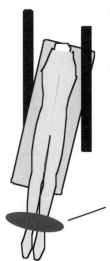

weight pad

Seated rowing (latisssimus dorsi, biceps)
Grab bar on Universal machine with underhand grip, keeping elbows close to your body and slightly bent with arms extended. Remember to keep your back straight, chest open, and shoulders back.

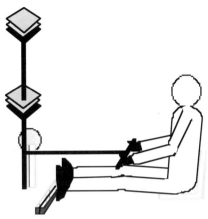

Pull the bar toward your navel, still keeping your elbows in. Then allow the bar to return in controlled fashion.

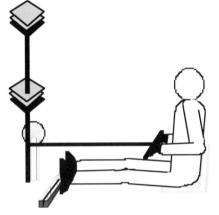

Shoulder shrug (optional)
(trapezius, rhomboids)
Hold a free weight with your arms extended down and your hands shoulder width apart. Start with your shoulders dropped forward and down. Looking straight forward, pull your shoulders up and back, opening your chest. Roll your shoulders back down, controlling the weight.

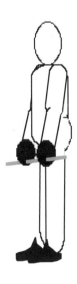

Calf raises (gastrocnemius and soleus)

With your feet flat on the ground, support a free weight on your shoulder—without resting it directly on your neck. Raise up on your toes and return with control. You can also do this one leg at a time standing on the edge of a step or calf board without a weight.

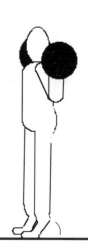

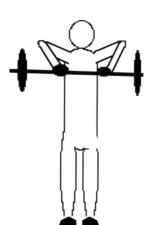

Upright rows
(deltoids, trapezius, biceps)

Start with your arms extended down to your waist, grasping a free weight with your hands at shoulder width. Raise the bar to chin level, keeping your elbows above the bar, and return to waist level with control.

Triceps extension
(triceps, latissimus dorsi)

Start bent over with back straight, both ams hanging down to a bench. Hold a dumbbell in one hand and support your weight with the other. Pivot the arm with the weight backward and upward to hip level. Remember to keep your elbow and knees slightly flexed.

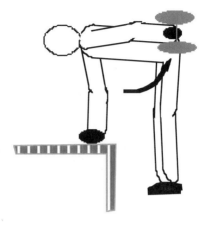

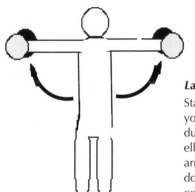

Lateral raises (deltoids, trapezius)
Stand with your back straight and your arms at your side holding a dumbbell in each hand. Keeping your elbows and knees flexed, raise your arms away from your body (palms down) to shoulder height. Lower with control.

Finish your program with some abdominal crunches, as described in numbers 2 and 3 of the five-minute fitness plan (pages 38 and 39).

5. ♥

Motivation

Osteoporosis is a thinning of bones often found in older people.

Y ou may have heard people say that exercise is its own reward, or that their day isn't complete unless they've had their workout. If you're not a regular exerciser or if your earlier attempts at exercise were more of a chore than a pleasure, you might find it hard to understand what motivates some people to exercise. In this chapter, we'll try to explain some of the underlying factors in body chemistry and psychology that not only encourage people to exercise but make it fun. Along the way, we'll continue our theme of encouraging you to move beyond the five-minute workout to a lifestyle of wellness.

Put yourself into the picture for a moment at the end of an exercise session. Feel the warmth of your muscles. Your body relaxes and your mind is clear. Your senses are heightened and you are conscious of every sound, sight, smell, and touch. Your eyes gleam and your skin glows. You take a shower or a soak, and your good mood follows you throughout the day. Friends or family comment on how well you look. You are creative and able to concentrate when you are working. Petty annoyances roll off and fail to dampen your spirits. At the end of the day, sleep comes easily and is restful.

Intellectually, you also know that your body and mind are becoming stronger, and your prospects for a healthy life are improved. Your chances of developing such degenerative diseases as osteoporosis and heart disease are reduced. In short, the quality of your life has been enhanced by exercise.

That is the motivation for exercising, its ultimate payoff. Not only is it fun to engage in an activity that you enjoy, but you are gaining health benefits.[1] Remember also that although we have been describing a relatively extensive exercise program of aerobics and lifting, studies repeatedly show that moderate exercise, like walking, has a great benefit. In fact, it appears that a program of overly strenuous exercise is a "de-motivator" and causes people to drop out of exercise programs.

Lise Gauvin, for instance, found substantial differences in four groups of individuals with regard to exercise.[2] The first group, whom she called "autonomous exercisers," were committed to attaining health and fitness, and they took the attitude that their lives depended on exercise. They typically exercised at about a 75-percent intensity, which could be termed "comfortably hard," but they truly enjoyed doing it. Another researcher, George Sheehan, also looked at autonomous exercisers and found that their minds are working on other subjects—family or work, for instance—or are often not focused on anything at all.[3] But their thinking is separate from the exercise program. He found that these people get out of sorts and feel that they are missing something when they do not work out.

In contrast, Gauvin's second group, fitness-program exercisers, relied more on a friend to keep them participating and didn't really like the exercise. They were more likely to focus directly on the exercise and pushed themselves to the hard range of intensity. After their workouts, they felt fatigued rather than energized.

The third group identified by Gauvin was fitness-program dropouts. They had exercised in the very hard range and were preoccupied with not stopping their program—until they gave up completely. Finally, the fourth group, sedentary individuals, think that exercise should be fun but doubt that it ever could be. They have any number of reasons for not exercising, including the amount of time that has to be committed to it.

The exercise program we have outlined in the first four chapters of this book is designed to help you become an autonomous exerciser and to avoid the pitfall of pushing too hard or engaging in an activity that you really don't enjoy. If you have been inactive, the best place to start is our five-minute workout. This program is neither exhausting nor painful, and you'll find that it's fun. As you feel the benefits of this simple program, we hope you'll be motivated to try other types of exercises.

What exercise is right for you? We aren't trying to "sell" you any particular exercise. You can walk and enjoy the outdoors, feeling the sun and breeze, smelling the flowers in the spring and the leaves in the fall. You can jog or run and get the same benefits of walking, plus cover more terrain and see different sights. You can bicycle and cover even more ground. A bike can even become your mode of transportation some days. One of the authors has an "around town" bike that takes her to errands on campus. The editor of this book has been bicycling to work (12-plus miles one way) for over 15 years. Swimming is a great exercise if your joints or back do not allow you to run. In all of these exercises, you get time to yourself, or you can share the time with a friend.

Skiing is just one of a myriad of activities that can benefit you. Many do not involve athletics—walking, gardening, and even doing housework are equally beneficial.

Even though most people would agree that regular physical activity is good for the body, mind, and spirit, it's hard for people to get started. We have mentioned that fact many times already and, indeed, that's why we tested the five-minute fitness program.

Let's look at the factors that hold people back

from starting an exercise program or that cause people to drop out:
- lack of time,
- inconvenience,
- interference from other responsibilities,
- too hard or too easy,
- discomfort with current body image,
- desire for quick results, and
- the perception that exercise is boring or no fun.

The five-minute program is designed with these reasons in mind. The exercises are not difficult, don't take much time, can be done on your own, and don't last long enough to be boring. While we hope you will build on the five-minute program, it will always be your backup, your buffer, your way of staying toned up—and your means of motivation.

You have to take the first step. The five-minute program may be the best thing going, but if you are not motivated to at least try it, all the suggestions we make in this book will be to no avail. We will be the first to agree that maintaining a regular exercise program and healthy eating habits requires considerable motivation.

The **intrinsic drive** to exercise comes from within you.

Individuals who are goal-oriented are more likely to carry out their commitment to physical exercise. The best motivation is an inner drive that almost compels you to exercise. Self-motivation does not come from outside. We can attempt to encourage you with our own enthusiasm for exercise, or we can attempt to share our concern that a sedentary lifestyle causes your body to deteriorate before its time. Neither of those approaches will work unless you feel the motivation to start. The beginning of that motivation is awareness—awareness of your hopes and dreams, and awareness of your body.

The best type of motivation is one that drives you toward a healthy lifestyle. If you are motivated to exercise or eat wisely because your best friend, significant other, or boss does, then your chances of maintaining your healthy lifestyle are much less than if you decide for yourself to do so.

A typical motivation for exercising is to lose weight because, for instance, your summer clothes don't fit or because your physician or insurance policy demands it. While weight loss is a valid goal of an exercise program, our concern is what happens after you reach your goal. The temptation would be to stop exercising. If your sole motivation is to lose ten pounds and then return to your former habits, exercise will seem more like a punishment and your motivation may be negative. If your goal is to enjoy exercise and develop a healthy lifestyle, the motivation is positive, exercise will be more natural, and the weight loss will come as part of the program.

Your body is designed for activity. Muscles need to be exercised for best functioning. Bones need exercise to remain strong and dense. Lungs and heart likewise need to be exercised regularly to maintain most efficient functioning.

The best motivation for exercise is the improvement in the quality of life. A regular exercise program gives you the stamina you need for a full day of sightseeing on vacation or for a last-minute dash through the airport to catch a plane. It gives you the ability to get through the day and maintain your productivity. It helps you meet the demands of job and family. And it even helps curb your appetite, or, at minimum, burn excess calories. Exercise and good health habits can change your life.

More than 30 years ago, psychologist Abraham

Maslow developed the concept of the hierarchy of human needs.[4] His idea was that a person would not progress to higher-level needs until the needs of the lower levels were satisfied and that people would try to satisfy their needs in a particular order. From bottom to top, the following are those needs:

1. *Physiological needs.* These involve basic survival factors (e.g., food, water, oxygen, and shelter).
2. *Safety needs.* Once a food supply is assured, a person will look for security, protection, avoidance of pain, and structure in the environment.
3. *Love needs.* On the next level, a person who is fed and feels secure will seek warm, satisfying relationships, affiliation, and affection.
4. *Esteem needs.* People who feel loved and have food and safety will seek recognition and self-respect, including confidence, independence, and attention and appreciation.
5. *Self-actualization.* Having achieved the other four categories, a person seeks self-fulfillment, becoming relatively independent from the environment and becoming all that he or she is capable of being.

Maslow argues that human beings have the capacity for a meaningful existence in which they fulfill their potential but they are prevented from achieving that potential because of conditions in the environment. Looking at the hierarchy, you can see the barriers to exercise. A person who is battling for food and safety cannot really consider the higher-level needs. If you're mired in one of the lower levels, it is hard to see your way to the self-actualization that is found in an exercise program.

Yet it is possible to remove at least some of the barriers once you recognize them. An exercise program, for instance, may initially fulfill your need for esteem. Our brief study gave an indication of such an effect. That probably is not enough to carry you forever, but when people have recognized that you are an exerciser you may continue because you have also found that exercise allows you to perform up to your potential. In fact, you may transcend your ego needs and become concerned with those of others.

Some people seem "addicted" to exercise, in a healthy way, and they speak of experiencing a "runner's high." This is probably the only case where an addiction can be a positive thing. In 1976, William Glasser developed the theory of positive addiction, which comes from inside.[5] While negative addictions, such as to drugs or alcohol, relieve the pain of failure and provide temporary pleasure (at a price!), positive addictions could lead to psychological strength, improved imagination, and creativity.

Glasser suggested that participating in such activities as yoga or vigorous exercise can lead to a positive addiction. We suggest that intense participation in any regular activity may lead to a positive addiction. When the body achieves the appropriate state, the imagination is freed, creativity improves, and your mind can develop more options for solving difficult or frustrating problems. Proof of positive addiction occurs with exercisers who are forced to neglect their habit for a time. They become guilty and anxious.

Glasser's idea of an appropriate activity is one that is noncompetitive, can be done easily without much mental effort, and can be done alone. The person should believe that the activity has mental, physical, or spiritual value, and that persisting allows improvement. He also said the exerciser should not be critical of his or her performance. His original idea was that the activity should be done for 40 to 60 minutes per day for at least six months.

During a runner's high or a positive addiction, a person may not be aware of events going on around her or him. If the person then quits exercising, he or she may experience a form of withdrawal. Unlike chemical addictions, this withdrawal is not harmful, but it is noticeable.

You probably won't experience a positive addiction during the five-minute exercise program, but we would like you to become hooked on exercise. Your body has a chemical basis for feeling good as a result of exercise. As you exercise, your pituitary gland produces pain-killing hormones called endorphins. Chemically similar to morphine, endorphins may be the source of runner's high and positive addiction. Since they are produced naturally in your body, they are not harmful. Exercising long enough to achieve a runner's high also promotes increased blood circulation, improved muscle tone, increased flexibility, and a more efficient exchange of oxygen and carbon dioxide in the body.

Endorphins are responsible for "runner's high."

Exercise-Success Gauge

Will you be successful in maintaining an exercise program? It is not always possible to tell who will stick with exercise, but the self-inventory in the box on the next page gives you an indication of how easy or difficult it might be for you to stay with an exercise program.

Score the inventory by adding together the seven numbers you circled. If your total score is 24 or less,

Table 1

Exercise-Success Inventory

For each statement circle the number underneath the letter that describes your reaction most closely. A= extremely uncharacteristic, B = somewhat uncharacteristic, C = neutral, D = somewhat characteristic, and E = extremely characteristic.

	A	B	C	D	E
1. I get discouraged easily.	5	4	3	2	1
2. I don't work any harder than I have to.	5	4	3	2	1
3. I seldom if ever let myself down.	1	2	3	4	5
4. I'm just not the goal-setting type.	5	4	3	2	1
5. I'm good at keeping promises, especially ones I make to myself.	1	2	3	4	5
6. I don't impose much structure on my activities.	5	4	3	2	1
7. I have a very hard-driving, aggressive personality.	1	2	3	4	5

Scoring: 25 or more—once you start, you'll probably be able to continue
24 or less—push hard and don't become discouraged

you may have to push yourself to exercise and fight the tendency to drop out.

Don't let this inventory be a self-fulfilling prophecy, however. The following are ways to increase the likelihood that you'll be able to start and continue exercising.

(1) *Make it fun.* Invite a friend, spouse, or partner to join you. Play your favorite tape (with appropriate exercises). Exercise in your yard on a warm day. Choose your best time of day for exercise to increase your efficiency and pleasure.

(2) *Visualize your muscles strengthening and your fitness level increasing.* After all, that is what is happening. Your chances for lower back pain will diminish, and those stronger muscles will help you with everyday tasks. Work and play will become easier.

(3) *Envision a new, firmer you.* Think of those favorite clothes that will fit comfortably and imagine how your appearance will improve.

(4) *Imagine a more confident, assertive, and positive you.* Imagine a calmer, happier you.

(5) *Make exercise a part of the time you set aside for personal renewal.* To reach the wellness level that you desire, it is important that you create time for renewal. During this personal time, people might take a long bath or a long walk, meditate, cook, read, or simply enjoy a few minutes of peace and quiet. When you set aside this personal time, make the five-minute workout a part of it.

(6) *Give yourself the proper rewards for exercise.* Rewards could be reading a book that you've been meaning to pick up, listening to some favorite music, or purchasing some clothes that you have long needed.

The best short-term reward, of course, is the improved muscle tone that you will achieve. Increased strength in arm and leg muscles means being more at ease in your everyday work and play. Increased strength means more endurance throughout the day and a long-term retardation of the aging process.

Getting into an exercise program and staying with it is a motivator in itself. That is the point of the five-minute fitness program. It's easy to start, and once you have started, it's easy to stay with. We hope that you will enjoy exercising and expand your program.

Long-term, your reward for a lifelong program of exercise and nutrition is wellness, a concept that we have mentioned briefly in this chapter. In the next chapter, we will delve more deeply into wellness and how it works for you. ❤

References

[1] See: S. N. Blair et al., "Physical Fitness and All-Cause Mortality: A Perspective Study of Healthy Men and Women," *Journal of the American Medical Association,* 262, No. 17 (1989), pp. 2395–2401; "Physical Activity and Psychological Benefits: A Position Statement," *International Journal of Sport Psychology,"* 23, No. 1 (1992), pp. 86–91; W.L. Haskell et al., "Cardiovascular Benefits and Assessment of Physical Activity and Physical Fitness in Adults," *Medicine and Science in Sports and Exercise,* 24, No. 6 (1992), pp. 201–220; C.C. Johnson and C. Slemneda, "Osteoporosis: An Overview," *The Physician and Sports Medicine,* 15, No. 11 (1987), pp. 65–68; C. Lenfant, "Physical Activity and Cardiovascular Health: Special Emphasis on Women and Youth," *Medicine and Science in Sports and Exercise,* 24, No. 6 (1989), pp. 191–210.

[2] L. Gauvin, cited in G. Sheehan, "Viewpoint: It's Easy to Stay Motivated When You Love What You Do," *Runner's World,* March 1992, p. 16.

[3] Ibid.

[4] A. Maslow, *Motivation and Personality* (New York: Harper, 1954).

[5] W. Glasser, *Positive Addiction* (New York: Harper & Row, 1976).

Glossary

Adrenaline—A body chemical that energizes and strengthens the system for immediate action.

Autonomous exercisers—People for whom exercise has become part of their routine.

Degenerative diseases—Conditions in which body functions are gradually impaired or lost, such as osteoporosis (thinning bones) and heart disease.

Endorphins—Body chemicals that produce soothing effects.

Hierarchy of human needs—A widely accepted theory that people who satisfy certain basic needs, such as food and safety, will then seek higher-level needs, such as love and esteem.

6.

Wellness

Wellness is far more than the absence of sickness. Wellness is a positive frame of mind—the feeling that we can solve any problem we might face and that we can control our fate. Wellness is loving ourselves and others. It is optimism, energy, and a strong sense of humanity and fair play. Wellness encompasses our ability to think, feel, communicate, connect, care, work and play, and experience the full range of emotions.

The concept of wellness encourages us to take responsibility for our own actions, health, and well being. By working toward wellness, we cease being passive or victimized and instead become assertive in solving our problems. We focus our thoughts and actions for the betterment of ourselves and others. We learn to solve problems when we can do so and to gracefully accept matters that we cannot influence. Wellness means that we strive to be fit physically and mentally, albeit without obsession.

The above explanation transcends the old definition of wellness as simply being physically fit. Many of us know athletes who are compulsive in their exercise or eating habits. They are physically fit, but they may not have achieved wellness, which also involves health in emotions and thoughts. Instead of eliminating stress from their lives they may well have increased their stress levels—and those of the people with whom they work or live. If they cannot relate well to other people or to life in general, their physical fitness has not become wellness.

In fact, wellness does not require complete physical functioning. Persons with physical challenges who have transcended those challenges probably have a greater degree of wellness than a person who com-

Wellness is far more than just physical fitness.

pulsively runs marathons or lives an otherwise unbalanced life. Physical challenges do not automatically prevent a person from achieving wellness. In this chapter, we will discuss the components of wellness and explain why wellness is important.

Components of Wellness

We all know people who seem perpetually optimistic and upbeat about situations that would send others into deep depression. Their secret may be wellness. Milton wrote: "The mind is its own place, and in itself can make a heaven of hell, a hell of heaven." That's a key to the secret of wellness. The ability to resist illness and depression in the face of adversity is termed "hardiness" by researchers. Hardiness, as defined by Suzanne Kobasa, for instance, is "a set of beliefs about oneself, the world, and how they interact. It takes shape as a sense of personal commitment to what you are doing, a sense of control over your life, and a feeling of challenge."[1]

Kobasa adds that the attributes that contribute to hardiness or wellness seem to be commitment, control, and challenge.[2] Being committed implies long-term goals and a desire to affect the outcome of events in a positive manner. Commitment gives one a sense of purpose, a reason to be, and something to which to aspire. It requires focus, endurance, and planning.

Autonomy is being able to make one's own decisions and control one's activities.

Time and again, health researchers have realized that people who believe that they have some control over illnesses, even terminal illness, either recover more quickly or survive longer than those who feel helpless and dependent.[3] Individuals who have more autonomy in their job have fewer illnesses than those who do not.[4] Control is the belief that you can cushion the blow of a circumstance by the manner in which you view and react to it.

The belief that you control your own behavior promotes health. It leaves you with the conviction that even though events around you may deteriorate, you will remain well.[5]

Challenges provide us with goals, cultivate an innate desire to win, and instill us with the ambition to try harder and to achieve in spite of great odds. Healthy people seem to welcome challenges.[6] Rather than view a task as drudgery, these people see their work as an opportunity and look forward to finding solutions and improving their performance. People who find challenges pleasant don't seem to notice the negative aspects of such situations and cherish the journey as much as the destination.

Becoming Healthy and Happy

In the last chapter we discussed runner's high and the role of endorphins. Certainly exercise is one of the keys to becoming healthy and happy. Avram Goldstein suggests that endorphins are produced not only in reaction to exercise but to such things as beautiful music, scenery, or artwork; scenes from a movie, play, ballet, or book; sexual activity; moments of nostalgia, high inspiration, or sudden insight; and success in a competitive endeavor. But wellness extends far beyond endorphins.[7]

Self love. The keystone of personal wellness is self love. This is not vanity or placing oneself over other people or the rest of creation. It is also not selfishness, which is often confused with self love. Selfishness implies looking after one's own welfare at the expense of others and without concern for others. In contrast, self love means taking care of ourselves physically and mentally so that we may in fact give more of ourselves to friends, family, colleagues, and the world. If we do not take time out to take care of our own mental and physical needs, how can we contribute fully to the world?

Developing wellness means that we must set aside time for ourselves—to contemplate our own feelings and needs and to exercise our bodies and minds. Talk to a friend, listen to music, do what you want—this time belongs to you. The greatest problem experienced by people suffering from stress is not having enough time for themselves. The issue of time is the key theme of this book. If you have started on the five-minute fitness program, you know that you can find time if you decide to do so. It's a matter of making time a priority.

Relationships with Others

All of us need other people. Recognizing our need for belonging, participating, and feeling needed by others is an important step in wellness.[8] Developing mutual trust, respect, and love is crucial. If you have been busy with your career and family responsibilities, you may have brushed aside the rewards of deep relationships. Perhaps you have inadvertently lost the rich relationship you once had with your spouse or life partner. Although we sometimes have difficulty realizing it, relationships are one of the most important aspects of life. When couples in longtime marriages are asked what they think contributed to the success of their relationship, a frequent answer is that they are not only lovers but best friends. Unfortunately, many of us realize the importance of relationships only after they are severed by death.

Now is a good moment to set time aside to rees-

Reestablish a relationship now.

tablish relationships. We suggest that you take the first step. Call the person who means the most to you and set a date to get together. The cause of the separation is not important, but the relationship *is* important. Suggest a "getaway" weekend for your spouse or partner. As strange as it may seem, perhaps your spouse needs courting all over again. Building or rebuilding those relationships is part of the road to wellness.

Relationships with Community

It is equally important that we establish ties with our community and be aware of the world around us. A truly well person will understand local and national issues and vote on them. Wellness also involves wise use of earth's resources, avoiding waste and rejecting products that produce pollution.[9] By becoming aware of the issues of global wellness, you can contribute in your own way and avoid using up more of the earth's resources than you need. While not all of us can be dedicated to a cause, becoming involved with a civic project or volunteering our time to any one of the many civic organizations gives us a sense of a higher purpose, as well as another outlet for our creative energies.

One of the great prescriptions for loneliness or depression is to get involved. Volunteering is a great way to begin.

Exercise

You need not be an elite athlete to reap the benefits of exercise.[10] We have dedicated considerable space in this book to this facet of wellness. Exercise can involve many activities during your day, and not just your exercise program. Walk the stairs, for instance, rather than wait for an elevator. Stretch at your desk.

Pace the floor while you are thinking or talking on the telephone. Walk down the hall for coffee or water.

When you do exercise, remember to try different activities from time to time. Take advantage of the seasons, with cross-country skiing in the winter and swimming in the summer, for example. Learning to enjoy and appreciate the seasons is certainly an aspect of wellness.

Balance

Balancing work, play, and commitment to family and friends is not always easy. The wellness strategy is to decide on the amount of time alloted to each commitment and then be firm about participating in each activity as you have planned it. Set aside time for family and friends, to feed the relationships that are so essential.

We are not prescribing a particular balance or time allocation. It is fashionable to criticize workaholics, but many of us know some exciting people who fit this category. The key is whether the workaholic is a happy, productive person who has established some kind of balance involving relationships and play, in addition to work.

Taking time to play allows us time for relaxation and gives us perspective on our life, work, and problems. Like exercise, play can take many forms. It can be an exercise session with a close friend or family member. It can be a family gathering or it can be a session of reading a good book. No matter how you live or what your philosophy of work is, schedule some play.

The Workplace

Wellness is important in your workplace, whether you are an employee, supervisor, manager, or company owner. The chief threat against wellness in the workplace is stress, especially the stress that comes from not being appreciated. No matter how much or how often you work out, if your work life is stressful or if you feel unappreciated you will feel uncomfortable and you may be prone to illness.

Some bosses create stress in their employees through their treatment of people or their actions.[11] Financial rewards cannot make up for being given little or no credit for a job well done, for instance, or for being criticized unduly. Feeling unable to respond or retaliate, an employee often suffers in silence. This is a prescription for illness—at worst heart disease or stroke and at minimum many missed days.

If this describes your workplace, your health may be at stake. Here are three options for such a case. **(1)** If you can approach your supervisor, talk over your feelings and see what you can do to improve your standing. If you have an enlightened supervisor, you might convince her to introduce stress-management and wellness classes for employees and managers. **(2)** Look for work elsewhere. Even if you do not take another job, the search can be therapeutic. **(3)** Attend stress-management workshops and use the techniques you learn there. Later in this chapter we will touch on some stress-reduction activities. Inherent in each of these options is the concept of wellness—taking control of your situation and refusing to be a victim.

Psychoneuroimmunology

This immense word denotes the idea that your mind maintains power over your body's ability to resist or recover from disease. It is true that people who suffer from unrelieved stress are also more susceptible to disease. As teachers on a college campus, we

Your brain has power over your body's health.

find that students are more likely to become ill at midterm and final-exam time. These students are not using illness as an excuse to escape from the tests. Instead, they are unable to mitigate the stress of studying for exams and finishing their papers and projects all at once.

Many authors have written of the mind-body connection, including Norman Cousins, Deepak Chopra, and Bernie Siegel.[12] These authors have experienced and written extensively about the power of positive thinking, a philosophy developed by the late Norman Vincent Peale. These authors carry Peale's theories even further to suggest that the mind controls the body's immune system.

Evidence is collecting in support of extensive interaction between the nervous and immune systems.[13] The studies indicate that happy people are more likely to avoid colds, influenza, and perhaps even more serious diseases. Many health officials claim that over 70 percent of doctor visits are psychologically based. The mind-body connection is part of wellness.

Stress Management

Let's return now to that great enemy, stress. The chronic stressors for most of us are relationships, finances, and work. Ironically, most of us can deal reasonably well with crises and acute problems, while debilitating stress can come from nagging problems that don't seem to go away.[14] When you cannot deal with a situation, your body is stressed.

Stress develops from a bodily mechanism called the "flight or fight" reaction. In earlier millennia, people who faced a problem, say, the threat of a wild animal, could resolve it immediately by fighting it or fleeing from it. The body gears up for the situation by producing adrenaline, and increasing blood sugar and lipids.

Lipid is another word for fat.

Such arousal was a survival mechanism for primitive humans, but it's rarely useful in today's stressful situations, particularly those that create continual discomforts and from which there is no easy relief. Usually there is no way to lash out at these problems or to run from them, and there is no release from a repeated dose of hormones and other stress-related chemicals in your body.

Dealing with Stress

The first step in dealing with stress is to assess whether some or all of the stress is self-imposed. Current thought on stress management is that stress is partially in the "eye of the beholder."[15]

How a person perceives stressful situations is important in managing stress. For instance, research on restaurant managers found that the managers whose beliefs centered on perfectionism experienced exacerbated stress and burnout.[16]

If stress has you tied up in knots, here's some suggestions for unwinding.

If at least some stress is self-imposed, the theme to follow is one of having control over emotions and reactions to the stress. Once again, this is a matter of continuing to feel in control of our lives. It is impossible to avoid stress entirely. In fact, Hans Selye, an early stress researcher, points out that stress is a necessary element in life and that there is both good and bad stress.[17] Good stress helps you make deadlines and stimulates your creative powers. In short, it helps you to achieve. Good stress comes, for example, from enjoying successful relationships, rearing children, winning a sporting event, or writing a book. Good stress does drain your reserves, but recovery is quick and leaves you healthy. In contrast, long periods of frustration and bitterness can be debilitating.

Meyer Friedman invented the term "type A" for a person who is in a constant whirlwind of stress.[18] These people are impatient and have a driving need for accomplishment at the expense of their health and, perhaps, that of others. Subsequent researchers found that some type-A people are happy because they thrive on being busy and involved, while other type As are angry, hostile, and frustrated. The second group is more prone to the heart attacks that are connected with type-A behavior.

Self-Esteem and Stress

Control over stress seems to come from optimism, self-confidence, belief in yourself, and a fighting spirit. High self-esteem helps a great deal in combating stress. You can start to improve your self-esteem by lightening up on yourself and laughing at your own shortcomings. We need to be aware that everyone suffers from lack of self-esteem from time to time. Ironically, individuals who irritate us most with their braggadocio may suffer from self-esteem lower than ours.

Look at specific areas that concern you. If you feel, for example, that others don't listen to you, you could take a course in communications or read more about subjects that interest you. Be a careful listener while the other person is speaking instead of thinking about what you want to say next.

Exercise, good grooming, and achievement all seem to build self-esteem. As we have mentioned in previous chapters, exercise produces a sense of accomplishment and increases your sense of well being. Likewise, looking your best makes you feel good about yourself. Finally, be justly proud of your achievements. Eleanor Roosevelt is credited with saying that no one can make you feel bad about your abilities unless you let them.

Stress Proofing

The first line of defense for stress is to plan ahead. If you have a particularly difficult or long assignment or one that makes you nervous, work on it ahead of the deadline. Know the topic so well that your confidence grows. Plan your work so that you can get plenty of rest and relaxation as you work. Also plan activities to release your creative powers.

If certain people seem to stimulate stress in you, analyze the situation. If you cannot avoid them, perhaps you can befriend them. If certain situations create stress, learn to recognize them. Make a list of what is important to you and what is not important. Make sure not to overload yourself with duties, especially those that are not important. Complete your tasks according to the list you made. Then reserve some of your time for friends and family.

Another way to avoid stress is to come to terms with life. If your stress results from frustration with your or others' imperfections, realize that no one is perfect. Moreover, perfectionists rarely accomplish much. While you should take pride in your work and make it as good as you can, it is better to complete the assignment in a timely fashion and move on. Perfectionists often have many projects waiting for enough time to start them or the right time to finish them. In reality, nothing gets done in that situation.

Releasing Stress

Despite your best efforts, stress will build up from

time to time. You will find many books and articles that suggest methods of dealing with stress, including controlled breathing, relaxation, guided imagery, meditation, biofeedback, and exercises. We suggest that you use several of these techniques or combinations. For instance, if you are having difficulty releasing anger and frustration, relaxation techniques may work best after exercise. Or a good workout may offer you your best release. A long walk in fresh air almost always reduces stress. If you are more practiced with stress control, consider breathing and relaxation exercises in combination with imagery. Simple yoga postures combined with deep breathing may be useful.

For a relatively quick method of attacking stress, try the following:

Sit or lie in a quiet, dim room in a position most comfortable to you. Wear loose clothes, remove your shoes, and close your eyes. Take a deep breath, filling your lungs and chest. Slowly release the air. Repeat, breathing more deeply and slowly in a relaxed fashion. While breathing, tense and gradually relax all your muscles, beginning with the top of your head and progressing to the tips of your toes. Take your time—ten minutes or more—and repeat some muscles if necessary.

When you feel more relaxed, think of your favorite, peaceful place and imagine you are there. Some people imagine a sunny day and they are reading a book under a shade tree; others imagine sitting next to a waterfall; still others are in a wooded vale where birds are singing.

Sit quietly and allow yourself to come slowly back to reality. You should feel more relaxed and confident and ready to return to your work or to accomplish the task at hand. When you encounter anger or frustration, return mentally to that favorite place you found so relaxing.

Stressing Wellness

Controlling and managing stress may be one of the most important facets of wellness. Stress poisons our outlook on life and spoils even those activities that are usually fun or entertaining. With stress under control, wellness is within your reach. Being well allows you to empathize and communicate with others. It puts you in touch with your feelings, which, in turn, encourages you to respect and care for yourself in the most unselfish of ways.

Being well encourages creativity in work and play. It makes us want to rise in the morning full of energy and gives us the eagerness to start the day with a sense of adventure. It allows you to sleep well and peacefully at night with the sense that you have put forth your best effort for the day and will be able to do the same the next day.

Being well puts you in charge of your mind and body. It makes aging a pleasant experience, rather than a situation filled with the dread of disease or disability. Finally, being well allows us to smell the flowers and to use our senses and sensuality no matter what our profession, age, income, gender, race, athletic ability, or interests. In short, wellness means that the best things in life truly are free.

We have been discussing the importance of balance in your life as a part of wellness. In the next chapter, we will discuss another aspect of wellness—appropriate nutrition. Just as enjoying life is part of wellness, so is enjoying food. ❤

References

[1] Suzanne Kobasa, "How Much Stress Can You Survive?," *American Health,* September 1984, pp. 71–71.

[2] Ibid.

[3] R.E. Flannery, "Toward Stress-Resistant Persons: A Stress-Management Approach to the Treatment of Anxiety," *American Journal of Preventive Medicine,* 3, No. 1 (1987), pp. 26–40.

[4] T. Edward Hannah, "Hardiness and Health Behavior," *Behavioral Medicine,* Summer 1988, pp. 59–62.

[5] J. Rodin, "Aging and Health: Effects of Sense of Control," *Science,* 233 (1986), pp. 1271–1276.

[6] D. Diamond and M. Golin, "Dare to Love Your Job," *Men's Health,* June 1991, p. 85–87.

[7] Avram Goldstein, "Thrills in Response to Music and Other Stimuli," *Physiological Psychology,* 8, No. 1 (1980), pp. 126–129.

[8] B.Q. Hafen, K.J. Frandsen, R.J. Karren, and K.R. Hooker, "Social Support, Relationships, and Health" (pp. 255–282), and "Marriage and Health" (pp. 311–328), in *The Health Effects of Attitudes, Emotions, and Relationships* (Provo, UT: EMS Associates, 1992).

[9] R.E. Kime, *Wellness: Environment and Health* (Guilford, CT: Dishkin Publishing, 1992).

[10] S.N. Blair et al., "Physical Fitness and All-Cause Mortality: A Prospective Study of Healthy Men and Women," *Journal of the American Medical Association,* 262, No. 17 (1989), pp. 395–401.

[11] K. Pelletier and R. Lutz, "Healthy People—Healthy Business: A Critical Review of Stress Management in the Workplace," *American Journal of Health Promotion,* 23, No. 3 (1988), pp. 5–12.

[12] See, for example: Joan Borysenko, *Minding the Body, Mending the Mind* (New York: Addison-Wesley, 1987); Norman Cousins, *Head First: The Biology of Hope* (New York: E.P. Dutton, 1989); and Bernie Siegel, *Love, Medicine, and Miracles* (New York: Harper and Row, 1986).

[13] Pelletier and Herzing, pp. 27–56.

[14] D.A. Giordano, G.S. Everly Jr., and D.E. Dusek, *Controlling Stress and Tension: A Holistic Approach* (Englewood Cliffs, NJ: Prentice-Hall, 1990).

[15] H. Benson, *The Relaxation Response* (New York: Avon, 1975); and Hafen et al., pp. 255–282.

[16] V. Apte and M.H. Tabacchi, "Le Stress des Managers Hôteliers," *ESPACES*, No. 124 (November-December 1993), pp. 9–14.

[17] Hans Selye, *Stress Without Distress* (New York: J.B. Lippincott, 1974).

[18] M. Friedman and R.H. Rosenman, *Type A Behavior and Your Heart* (New York: Alfred A. Knopf, 1974).

Glossary

Autonomy—Making one's own decisions and controlling one's activities.

Lipids—Fats.

Psychoneuroimmunology—The concept that the mind has considerable control over a person's physical health.

Stroke—An interruption of blood to the brain that often causes lasting damage and loss of function.

Type-A behavior—A lifestyle of high pressure and quick action often thought to be connected to heart attacks.

7. ♥

Nutrition: You Are What You Eat

Enjoying food and beverage is one of life's great pleasures, and eating is part of health and fitness. This chapter offers a healthy approach to food—discussing ways to improve your nutritional approach and enjoy food. Imagine eating until you are full. Imagine pastas, pizzas, stir fries, seafood, steak, baked potatoes, and tantalizing fresh fruits and vegetables—even wine, beer, and spirits in moderation. If the key to good mental health is moderation, food is no exception. You certainly can enjoy the flavors, aromas, and textures of well-prepared foods in moderate portions. When your life is in balance and your fitness program in place, your appetite will be balanced as part of that lifestyle. A balanced approach to food can lower your risk of degenerative diseases and enhance your internal and external beauty.

Dietary Guidelines

Students, colleagues, and friends often suggest to us that healthy eating is too complicated. They don't know which writer, diet book, or television talk show to believe. It seems easy to get tangled in conflicting information.

In reality, the government's recommendations to the public for a healthy diet have changed little since 1978, when the U.S. Senate's Select Committee on Nutrition and Human Needs published dietary goals for the United States. Those same goals were published again in 1988 by the U.S. Department of Health and Human Services, and they were part of the Surgeon General's Report on Nutrition on Health.[1]

Those dietary goals have been translated into various forms of dietary guidelines from 1979 through 1992, when the latest version of the food pyramid was issued. The goals and guidelines have been consistent on several points: eat a variety of foods; consume plenty of fruits, vegetables, and grain products; limit fat and cholesterol intake; maintain a healthy weight by consuming moderate amounts of calories; consume sugar and salt in moderation; and drink alcohol in moderation if at all.[2]

The current food-group plan or food pyramid adds four more points to those longstanding recommendations. They are to eat moderate amounts of protein, maintain adequate calcium intake, avoid taking dietary supplements beyond the recommended daily allowance (USRDA), and maintain an optimal intake of fluoride.[3]

A note on USRDAs:[4] These recommended daily amounts of various nutrients apply to most normal, healthy people who are facing typical environmental stresses. The USRDAs are recommendations, not requirements, and they are certainly not minimum requirements. The USRDA amount includes a substantial extra margin of safety that provides for individual variations both in people's needs and in nutrient contents from various food sources.

In May 1994 the USDA required a change in the labeling of all FDA-regulated products and processed foods from USRDAs to "daily reference values" (RDV) and "reference daily intakes" (RDI). Although the values of the RDVs and RDIs are nearly the same as the former USRDAs, the USDA believes that consumers will gain more information

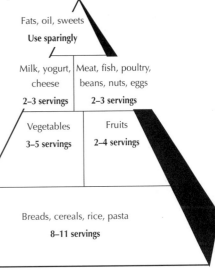

The USDA food pyramid stresses the value of nutrient-dense foods, such as breads and pasta, and fruits and vegetables.

from the new standards. Indeed, the required label on cans and other processed or regulated products now emphasizes the most important nutrients contained in food: carbohydrate, dietary fiber, sugar, and protein, as well as such items as fat, saturated fat, cholesterol, and sodium. The new RDVs are based on a 2,000-calorie diet, one that researchers now believe is appropriate for most women middle age and older.

While no one discounts the need for vitamins and minerals, the new labels do not emphasize them because eating a variety of foods, as suggested by the dietary guidelines, is most likely to ensure that a person consumes more-than-adequate amounts of these micronutrients. While we are aware of the public's and some scientists' interest in the so-called "anti-oxidant" nutrients, we believe that it is important to obtain them through food. Because food chemists still do not know the entire nutrient content of foods, taking pills in place of fresh, healthy food is neither desirable nor particularly safe.

Many people are worried about getting enough of the RDAs. Individuals often worry that they are not getting enough of a certain vitamin or mineral because they are not meeting the RDA each day. These people often resort to dietary supplements. We suggest that you take the approach to diet that we describe in this chapter.

The basic idea of **nutrient density** is to gain the greatest possible nutrition from a given amount of food.

Nutrient Density

The more a food resembles the original, farm-grown product, the more nutritious it is likely to be. That runs counter to the expectation that processed foods with added vitamins and minerals are high in nutrients. However, the fresher a food, the greater its nutrient density, which is defined as the amount of nutrients a food supplies in relation to the calories it contains. The higher the level of nutrients and the fewer the number of calories, the more nutrient dense a food is. For example, half a cup of ice cream contains the same number of calories as a whole cup of low-fat, plain yogurt and considerably more calories than a cup of skim milk. The milk and yogurt supply more calcium, protein, and riboflavin than does the ice cream. Therefore, the milk and yogurt are more nutrient dense than the ice cream.

A good comparison of nutrient density comes from the potato and its related products. A plain potato contains, among other things, 25 milligrams of vitamin C (one-half of the RDA) and less than one-tenth gram of fat. An equal amount of french fries (in terms of calories) contains only 7 milligrams of vitamin C and 10 grams of fat. The same amount of potato chips contains a mere 3 milligrams of vitamin C and 13 grams of fat. Needless to say, the whole potato contains considerably more dietary fiber than either the fries or the chips and is more nutrient dense than either processed product.

Serving Size

One of the greatest difficulties in attempting to follow nutrition guidelines is understanding serving or portion size. Dietary guidelines, nutrition information, and RDAs are generally given according to portion size. Sometimes it is hard to determine what a portion is. For instance, the U.S. Department of Agriculture defines a serving of meat, poultry, or fish as being about three ounces (after cooking). Restaurants typically serve six to eight ounces, and a common home serving is five or six ounces. Most nutrient charts, however, are based on the three-ounce serving. Consequently, people can ingest considerably more calories than they expect. This problem is magnified with such foods as cakes, pastries, or high-fat items such as butter, oils, cheese, processed or fatty meats, and deep-fried foods.

To ensure that you consume an appropriate and balanced amount of food, your diet should be based on serving sizes. Each component of your diet is given according to the number of servings in a day. As an example of how this works, we'll discuss how to build a nutritious diet using the food groups.

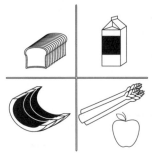

The current food pyramid is an excellent food guide, because it discourages fats, oils, and sweets and encourages only moderate intake of dairy foods and meat, poultry, fish, eggs, and nuts. The current guidelines emphasize our need for fruits, vegetables, and complex carbohydrates containing fiber. In the following section, we'll discuss a typical day's consumption, using the food pyramid as a guide.

Assembling a daily diet of nutritious food is made easy by keeping a rough tally of the number of servings from each food group.

For breakfast you could have one ounce of high-fiber, ready-to-eat cereal (about 3/4 cup) or half a cup of cooked cereal (1 serving of bread-cereal) and a slice of toast (1 more serving). You could have a half grapefruit or six ounces of juice (more than 1 serving of fruit) and a small banana (1 more serving), plus 1/2 cup of skim milk (1/2 serving) on your cereal.

Lunch could be 1/2 cup of black bean soup (1 serving of the meats-beans group) with a slice of whole-grain bread (1 serving of bread-cereal), plus 3 ounces of carrot sticks (1 serving), an orange (1 serving), and a cup of skim milk.

For dinner you could enjoy paella made with 2 or 3 ounces of fish (1 serving) over 3/4 cup of rice (1 1/2 servings), accompanied by three medium rolls

(3 servings), 3/4 cup of fresh cooked broccoli (1 1/2 servings of vegetables), and 1 ear of corn (1 more serving of vegetables), plus a sliced tomato as a salad (1 serving).

Dessert or a later snack could be oatmeal crunch (oatmeal over fruit topped with yogurt) or 1/2 an apple, 1/2 ounce cheese, and three or four crackers. Either one gives you 1/2 serving of bread-cereal, 1/2 serving of fruit, and 1/2 serving of dairy.

Tallying your intake for the day, you have consumed 8 servings of bread-cereal, 2 servings of meats-beans, 2 servings of dairy, nearly 4 servings of fruit, and 4 servings of vegetables. If you were careful in your use of butter, margarine, and oils, this day's consumption was just 1,600 calories.

Taking the example a step further, if you are at all active with jogging or "power walking," say 1/2 hour each day, you will burn 300–400 of those calories. Notice the absence of "diet" or synthetic foods in this example—and there will be no feelings of food deprivation.

Now, you do not have to carry this book with you to remind you of serving sizes when you are in the grocery store or the kitchen. On the back of each food package is the nutrition-facts label that gives you the serving size, the number of servings in the container, and the food's contribution to the RDI or RDV of calories, protein, and other nutrients. The label also gives you information about the amount of sodium and fats contained in each serving of the food.

Your intake of fats, oils, and sugars should be limited. Although food chemists have yet to assess the relative value of "good" fats and "bad" fats, it is clear that too much of any fat does not contribute to your long-term health. On the other hand, eating no fat at all is also not a wise choice, unless one is under doctor's orders. Check your recipes and food labels to assess fat sources and see where fat can be reduced. There is, for instance, little reason to add oil to a vegetable-based soup; the fat in muffins can often be cut in half and it can be eliminated entirely in pancakes; and sugar and fat can usually be trimmed substantially in corn bread and other quick breads. One secret for baking cakes is to substitute apple-sauce for much of the fat in the recipe. Instead of sautéing vegetables in fat or oil, "sweat" them at a low temperature.

Butter versus margarine. A tablespoon of butter contains as much fat as a tablespoon of margarine. As studies are completed, it appears that one is in no way superior to the other. Use your favorite spread—in moderate amounts.

Balance

Your dietary target should be a balance of calories contributed by carbohydrates, fat, and protein. The best combination is a diet that provides 60–65 percent of calories from carbohydrates (preferably high in fiber), 25–30 percent from fat, and 10 percent from protein. To hit that protein target without exceeding the fat goal, one must choose lean meats and a complementary arrangement of legumes and grains, prepared without additional fats or oils. Pastas should be served with tomato or marinara sauces (watch for hidden fat), or with vegetable stir fries prepared with a minimum of oil. A secret of Chinese cooks is to start with a bit of oil, but then to add only enough water to keep the stir fry moist. If your pasta sticks together, try reduced chicken stock instead of oil to keep it from sticking.

Beating fat. There are many other ways to cut your dietary fat without sacrificing taste. We must recognize that our taste buds like fat. It adds flavor to foods and gives them "mouth feel" or a pleasing texture. The anti-fat trick is to fool your taste buds. You can, for instance, use 1-percent or skim milk on your breakfast cereal without any loss in taste. Buy low-fat or non-fat yogurt. When it's mixed with fruit, the flavor is just as good as the high-fat variety. Plain low-fat yogurt is an excellent substitute for sour cream on baked potatoes or burritos, and yogurt can be mixed with low-fat mayonnaise to add nutrition and cut calories in a spread. Try the European approach to cheese, as suggested in the sample day's food consumption above. Instead of eating a large amount as an appetizer, save it for after the meal and you won't consume as much. Taking another leaf from the Europeans, learn to enjoy fruits as dessert. Well-ripened fruit is as sweet as any confection, and it provides a bonus of fiber, vitamins, and minerals.

A word about alcohol: This chemical stimulates appetite and dulls judgment. Therefore, if you drink at all, wait to consume wine or beer with your meal rather than before. Sip slowly and savor the flavor. Wine, beer, or spirits can have a healthy place in your diet of moderation. Moreover, there is evidence that alcohol retards the clotting of blood in one's arteries. That is no reason to begin drinking if you do not consume alcohol, however. Your balanced diet that is low in fat and high in fiber will do more to protect your arteries than alcohol ever could.

About Fat

We mentioned that a no-fat diet is unwise, but there has been much confusion regarding the health ef-

Saturated fat, which has a high hydrogen content, has been linked to heart disease.

fects of saturated fat and dietary cholesterol. We will try to untangle some of that confusion.

Cholesterol. The role of dietary cholesterol in the evolution of heart disease remains under debate. Well-designed research in the 1970s suggested that blood cholesterol is boosted only somewhat by the consumption of cholesterol in healthy people. In essence, the research indicated that the consumption of saturated fats had a greater effect on blood cholesterol than did cholesterol intake. Nevertheless, people who have elevated levels of blood cholesterol (above 200 mg/dl) should restrict their dietary cholesterol, as well as their fat intake, as indicated by their physician.

Fats. Saturated fatty acids appear to be more of a threat than cholesterol. The dietary goals suggest consuming no more than 10 percent of our calories as saturated fat, up to 10 percent as polyunsaturated fat, and 10 percent as monounsaturated fats. Once again, the total amount of all fat should not exceed 30 percent of calories.

Nutrition and Food Behavior

The above discussion may seem complicated at first, but if you practice a bit the guidelines are easy to follow. Proper nutrition and eating well can be understood. Calorie charts, percentage of calories from fat, and serving sizes all make sense. But the fact remains that many people suffer from the effects of overnutrition—obesity, heart disease, cancer, and stroke. The difficulty lies in practice. Our heads tell us to eat healthily, but our emotions and our senses say otherwise.

Many factors influence our food behavior, including income, occupation, education, culture, religious beliefs, lifestyle, nutrition knowledge, family preferences, emotional needs, and even our genetic makeup.

Even though we know what it is to eat in a healthy fashion, many factors intervene to tempt us away from our efforts to consume foods that contribute to our continued good health. Understanding this point is essential to good health and a balanced approach to food. When you overindulge, as everyone does occasionally, don't be guilty. Food should be enjoyed. But if you fall into the trap of looking at food as good or bad, or count calories too religiously, you will lose your enjoyment of food.

It takes some willpower to develop and maintain good eating habits, but once you have achieved them you will wonder why you didn't do it sooner. You will enjoy the increase in energy, the improvement in your mental outlook, and the knowledge that you are doing the best for your health's sake.

When and Where to Eat

Start off with breakfast. A healthy breakfast is essential for the energy and concentration needed at work or at school. Breakfast is the ideal meal to obtain fiber, with high-fiber cereals, hot or ready to eat, and bananas or berries. That kind of breakfast gives you staying power till noon, especially if you top it off with additional fruit or fruit juice. In contrast, Danish pastries, sticky buns, donuts, or muffins heavy in fat or sugar can cause blood sugar to take a roller-coaster ride and stimulate hunger long before lunch.

In some societies, lunch is the major meal of the day. This was true in the United States when most of the work was manual labor. A large lunch is still a wise choice, so that you can avoid a starving sensation in midafternoon or when you arrive home from work. A simple, but effective lunch might be a sandwich, a bit of lean meat on whole-wheat bread, with yogurt and a piece of fruit or cut-up vegetables. Try to avoid burgers and fries, and above all, skip the so-called "diet plate" offered in so many lunch counters. One wonders how a hamburger patty with cottage cheese on the side came to be considered diet food!

Dinner time and afterward is the time when many Americans overeat, especially those who skip breakfast or lunch. People have a desire to snack while preparing dinner or while watching television. One way to avoid overeating is not to eat while watching TV, because it is easy to overeat while concentrating on something else. The delightful tradition of dinnertime conversation is another way to avoid overeating.

Eating slowly is a good approach to enhancing digestion and to cut down on overeating. Some experts believe it takes the brain 20 minutes to receive the signal that the stomach is full. Eating slowly allows that message time to penetrate. Moreover, a relaxed eating pace gives you time to concentrate on enjoying the flavor and texture of your food.

Weight Maintenance

One of the goals you may have for your exercise program is weight maintenance. How much we weigh is a result of many factors, some of them beyond our control, as we will discuss in a moment. Nevertheless, it is true that eating properly is one of the elements in weight control. Not only can we maintain a healthy weight, but we can gain energy and reduce our risk of disease by eating properly.

One of the keys to healthy eating is to avoid making yourself feel deprived. The reason that people cannot maintain the weight loss from most fad diets is that the dieter feels deprived of food he or she normally eats. We suggest that you not restrict the types of food you eat, but instead pay attention to the guidelines we just discussed for the food groups, particularly fat. If you have reached a healthy weight for your body type and you include regular aerobic exercise as part of your lifestyle, there is no reason that you cannot enjoy a bowl of ice cream, a rich brownie, or steak and french fries once in awhile. The goal is to hit your low-fat, low-sugar target about 90 percent of the time. This approach flows from our contention that enjoying food is part of wellness.

Weight maintenance was once little problem for most people. In days past, hard physical labor and a sometimes inadequate diet was the norm. Under those conditions, it was sometimes difficult to *gain* weight. Workers could easily consume and burn 4,000 calories a day. Now a petite-size woman could easily get by on 1,500–1,800 calories and a small, inactive man up to 2,200. A moderate to large-size woman who works out could consume and burn 2,200–2,800 calories a day and an active man could burn up to 3,500.

A key to weight management is to eat only when you are hungry. Never eat "by the clock," when others are eating, or just to pass the time. Don't force yourself to eat more food after you have reached your satiety level. No additional points are awarded for clean plates if you have eaten too much! Once the meal is over, food should be cleared away so there is no temptation to pick at the food and eat more than is necessary.

As you age, you will notice that it may be more difficult to maintain your weight. The trick is to increase your exercise level, and you may also want to trim your calorie level a bit. The real contribution to weight gain among middle-aged people is simply that they no longer are as active as when they were young. That's why we suggest building exercise into your schedule.

Stay happy. Recent research suggests that depressed or stressed people eat more than those in a good frame of mind. The use of food as a mood enhancer is unwise in the long run. Instead, search for calorie-free activities that boost your mood. We think aerobic exercise is one of the best choices.

It is easiest and healthiest to maintain your weight by consuming a diet high in complex carbohydrates and low in fat. Complex carbohydrates come from fruits, vegetables, grains, and legumes. Planning a meal around your favorite meat is fine, as long as you remember the serving-size guidelines and balance the meal with foods from other groups.

About salad. Many people think salad is a healthy part of a meal. It certainly is, provided that the salad is not just iceberg lettuce and that the dressing is low in fat. Iceberg and its lettuce cousins are 99-percent water and contain few nutrients. You can, of course, boost the nutrient value of your salad by adding broccoli, peppers, tomatoes, and the like. Brilliant green, yellow, red, and orange vegetables contain high amounts of beta-carotene (a nutrient connected with lower cancer risk), fiber, and vitamins and minerals. Salad dressings are the other pitfall in salad. Many dressings supply as much as

Beta-carotene, found especially in carrots and other orange vegetables, is changed to vitamin A in your body.

100 calories per tablespoon because of their fat content. A hamburger might contain less fat than a dollop of some salad dressings.

Diet products, such as colas, gelatins, puddings, and desserts, cannot help you lose weight, unless they are part of an overall healthful approach to weight maintenance. In fact, you may not need diet food at all if you use the nutrient-dense approach we have suggested here. Instead, by controlling your fat intake at most meals, you can eat the "real thing," as we have already explained.

Body Type

People come in all shapes and sizes. Your genetic makeup plays a large role in determining your physical appearance. The "set-point" theory suggests that each person has a specific body type. Take steps to go below that point and your body strives to maintain it. But genetics is not the whole story. People with a greater number of fat cells have a larger management challenge in maintaining their weight at a desired level than people whose bodies do not have such cells. Clearly there are environmental contributions to a person's size.

Regardless of a person's body type, genetic makeup, or environmental influences, one thing is clear: inactivity seems to encourage obesity. The hunger and appetite-control mechanism seems to work best in people who remain active.

This is not a book about weight loss, but you may have a personal goal of trimming a few excess pounds that have accumulated over the years. If you find your body resisting your efforts to reduce weight levels, the suggestions that you have already read in this book for diet and exercise will be helpful. You may, however, want to augment your workout program by adding enough exercise to burn, say, another 300 calories per day while at the same time trimming your calorie intake by another 300. This approach should give you the gradual weight loss that is most likely to be permanent.

We urge you to be happy with the body you have inherited. Learn to see your own beauty, and don't compare your appearance with the young, emaciated models you see in fashion magazines. Chances are that no one will notice your hip size (or whatever) if your personality shows your inner wellness. Once again, we emphasize that wellness is more than just a physical attribute.

Traveling

Maintaining your exercise and nutrition plan on the road is difficult and the likelihood of temptation is great. To start with, don't give up your exercise program while traveling. You may have to change activities, but you can continue exercising. Many hotels have fitness clubs or jogging or walking routes, and don't forget your travel fitness kit.

Most hotels and restaurants have added nutritious, tasty, low-fat items to their menus. If you find no such items, you can modify the existing menu items by requesting that entrées be served with sauces or dressings on the side or without salt. That way you can control the amount of high-calorie sauce in the serving. Most kitchens are set up for such special requests. If they are not, you are completely within your rights simply to excuse yourself and find another restaurant.

Restaurants that are truly customer oriented may well create menu items for you on the spot. In a speech at Cornell University, one restaurant company executive recalled a time when a customer ordered a fruit salad, even though there was no such thing on the menu. Using garnishes and items from other dishes, the restaurant created a fruit salad.

Myths and Misinformation

We cannot close this chapter on nutrition without addressing the many myths and misleading information purveyed by those who wish to sell you their products. In this section, we will dispel myths about sugar, supplements, ergogenic acids, fad weight-loss diets, "detoxifying" diets, and diet products.

Sugar. Although sugar has been vilified for years, scientists can find little evidence that sugar is actually harmful, except to your teeth. The chief problem with sugar is that it adds calories without nutrients. Contrary to the popular wisdom that it "wires" people, sugar and its fellow starches have a relaxing effect and, in the presence of a small amount of protein, encourage drowsiness.[5] Sugar is sugar, regardless of its form. Honey, molasses, jelly, and "raw" sugar have no more health benefits than refined sugar.

Supplements. Dietary supplements gained popularity in the early 1940s, when it was discovered that doses of cod-liver oil were beneficial in preventing rickets and night blindness. Over the intervening years, supplements that supply vitamins, minerals, and other substances have become big business. Contrary to legend, ingesting extra vitamins and minerals does not give people more energy. That comes from eating a balanced diet. Athletes can increase their endurance by carbohydrate loading, but not by taking supplements.

The strength of dietary supplements comes for people who are malnourished. In the case of cod-liver oil, the people who were helped had inadequate supplies of vitamin D, usually supplied by sunlight and now found in fortified fluid milk. For people eating the typical American diet and having normal nutritional needs, supplements are unnecessary.

One cannot take vitamin pills in place of breakfast or lunch. They don't contain all the nutrients necessary for an active day, and they don't contain the calories and fiber your body needs to function. Furthermore, vitamins work in concert with each other. Increasing the intake of one may increase or decrease your need for another. Even a chemist specializing in biochemical uses of vitamins cannot have the knowledge necessary to balance large doses of vitamin supplements.

The old tale that if one pill is good, two must be better is just that, an old tale. Excessive use of supplements is at best wasteful and at worst dangerous. High doses of water-soluble vitamins, such as vitamin C and folic acid, are merely excreted by your body. Yes, you flush them down the toilet! In contrast, excessive doses of the fat-soluble vitamins, such as A, D, and K, can be toxic because they build up in your body until they are put to use. As a final note on the dangers of supplements, amino-acid supplements and protein supplements can cause kidney damage.

Ergogenic acids. Companies that produce ergogenic acids claim that they improve athletic performance. To date, scientists have found little support for that claim. The hundreds of ergogenic-acid products on the market do nothing to boost energy. What does boost energy is the proper diet and training habits of an athlete.

Detoxifying diets. The scene of primary action of so-called detoxifying diets seems to be the colon. The colon's chief job, however, is to absorb water from the digestive product. The colon is not one of the body's detoxifying agents. The chief "detox unit" is the liver, with assistance from the kidneys and other glands. Detoxifying is an intricate biochemical process that has nothing to do with juice diets or fasting. In fact, the process relies on the healthy functioning and full energy of all the body's cells. Mystical treatments, fasting, and living only on juice may hamper the biochemistry of detoxification.

Even more ridiculous are the diets that call for separating foods from each other and eating them at various intervals throughout the day, to avoid having them "rot" in your intestines. Such diets are not harmful, but they are time-consuming. Your digestive system is designed to work simultaneously on thousands of nutrients and components at once. The claim that, for instance, fruits and vegetables should be eaten separately from each other or from other foods has no validity. This claim is sometimes complicated by the claim that the acidity of fruits does not combine well with other foods. Once again, your system is well-armed to digest fruits. In fact, once they are digested and absorbed fruits become basic and work as a buffer against acids.

Diet books. The thousands of diet books published in the past decade or two have made plenty of money for their authors. Gimmicky diets found in books like these might be effective in helping you lose weight, but none of them are particularly effective in maintaining weight. This is because a "diet" is an aberration from your normal activities. Go off the diet and you have difficulty maintaining your weight loss. If you struggle with this matter, as most folks do, see a dietitian. Most hospitals have dietitians on their wellness staff, and many dietitians in private practice can give you good advice to fit your special needs.

Diet products. Diet food—fat reduced, sugar removed, portion controlled—has likewise become a big industry. Yet for all the diet drinks, gelatin, puddings, salad dressing, and even ice cream sold and consumed, there has not been a notable decline in America's obesity levels, probably due to the decline in physical activity. Liquid shakes, for instance, really do work to help you lose weight, but they don't help you learn to eat properly. Portion-controlled entrées can help you lose weight because they are part of a method. But these expensive products are not essential to a weight-maintenance program, if you use a serving-size approach to calories.

There is no real substitute for good nutrition and sound eating habits. It's never too late to start building those good habits. As with the exercise program we described earlier, you can start small and build up until you have internalized a healthy diet.

To get you started, the next chapter sets up some food suggestions and recipes for a tasty, nutrition-filled menu with plenty of variety. ❤

References

[1] U.S. Senate Committee on Nutrition and Human Needs, *Dietary Goals* (Washington, DC: U.S. Government Printing Office, 1978).

[2] U.S. Department of Health and Human Services, *Surgeon General's Report on Nutrition and Health* (Washington, DC: U.S. Government Printing Office, 1988).

[3] U.S. Department of Agriculture and U.S. Department of Health and Human Services, *Nutrition and Your Health: Dietary Guidelines for Americans,* 3rd edition, Home and Garden Bulletin No. 232 (Washington, DC: U.S. Government Printing Office, 1990).

[4] U.S. Department of Agriculture, *Food Guide Pyramid,* Home and Garden Bulletin No. 249 (Washington, DC: U.S. Government Printing Office, 1992).

[5] National Research Council, *Recommended Dietary Allowances,* 10th edition (Washington, DC: National Academy Press, 1989).

[6] Paula Kurzweil, "Nutrition Facts," *FDA Consumer,* May 1993, pp. 22–27.

[7] National Research Council, *Diet and Health Implications for Reducing Chronic Disease Risk* (Washington, DC: National Academy Press, 1989); K. Glanz, A. Krystal, G. Sorensen, R. Palombo, J. Heimdinger, and C. Probart, "Development and Validation of Measures of Psychosocial Factors Influencing Fat- and Fiber-Related Dietary Behavior," *Preventive Medicine,* 22 (1992), pp. 373–387; J. Nash, "Eating Behavior and Body Weight: Physiological Influences," *American Journal of Health Promotion,* 1987, pp. 5–15; K.H. Duncan, J.A. Bacon, and R.L. Weinseir, "The Effects of High- and Low-Energy Diets on Satiety, Energy Intake, and Eating Time of Obese and Nonobese Subjects," *American Journal of Clinical Nutrition,* 37 (1983), pp. 763–67; C. Bouchard, "Genetic Factors in Obesity," *Medical Clinics of North America,* 73 (1989), pp. 67–83.

[8] B. Spring, "Carbohydrates, Tryptophan, and Behavior: A Methodological Review," *Psychological Bulletin,* 102, No. 2 (1987), pp. 234–256.

[9] National Research Council *Diet and Health Implications for Reducing Chronic Disease Risk* (Washington, DC: National Academy Press, 1989).

Glossary

Beta-carotene—A nutrient associated with orange-colored vegetables that is converted into vitamin A in the body.

Cholesterol—A waxy substance needed for proper body functions, but dangerous if it sticks to and clogs arteries.

Detoxifying diet—A false theory of nutrition based on misinformation.

Fat-soluble vitamins—Micronutrients that are stored in the body's fat cells until needed (e.g., vitamins A, D, and K).

Food groups—Groupings of related foods, for the purpose of assembling a balanced diet.

Food pyramid—A way of picturing the recommendation that people obtain the bulk of their calories from breads, grains, fruits, and vegetables (the base of the pyramid), while limiting meats, dairy, and fat (the top of the pyramid).

Monounsaturated fat—With a variant chemical formula, thought to be the fat least harmful to humans.

Nutrient density—The relationship of the amount of nutrition in a food to the calories supplied by that food. Foods nearest their natural state have the highest nutrient density.

Polyunsaturated fats—A form of fat thought to have fewer links to heart disease than saturated fat.

RDI (recommended daily intake)—A term instituted in 1994 for target amounts for each day's consumption of food nutrients, replacing USRDA.

RDV (recommended daily values)—Similar to RDV, another term for target amounts for each day's consumption of food nutrients, replacing USRDA.

Saturated fat—A substance linked to heart disease.

Serving size—One unit of a given food, used as a means to count the relative amounts of different food groups consumed in a day.

Set point—The theoretical "proper" weight established by a person's genetic and environmental influences. Efforts to gain or lose weight beyond the set point are often unsuccessful.

Supplements —Vitamin and mineral pills that purport to improve on a good diet or make up for a poor one.

USRDA (United States recommended daily allowance)— The term used starting in 1978 for recommendations from government agencies regarding target amounts for each day's consumption of food nutrients.

Water-soluble vitamins—Micronutrients that are not stored in the body but are excreted when in excess (e.g., vitamins B and C).

8.

A Week of Healthy Eating

About the recipes

We have tried to make the recipes on the following pages as short and simple as possible. Most of them can be assembled quickly, although a few would benefit from being prepared the day before or being marinated overnight. In fact, an easy way to cook is to chop, season, and marinate in advance.

These recipes are intended to make cooking short and simple and to provide you with ideas for wholesome foods that have low fat, moderate sodium, and modest calories. There are enough recipes here for seven full days—seven each of dinner, lunch, and breakfast.

We hope that these recipes will inspire you to create your own healthy meals. We have found that the best way to encourage people to eat healthily is to encourage them to reduce fat and sodium in their favorite recipes.

Perhaps some of these recipes will become favorites. We have trimmed fat and sodium in many recipes, for example, by seasoning rice and noodles with defatted low-sodium fish or chicken stock perked up with spices or herbs. In place of straight sour cream, we suggest a mix of non-fat yogurt and sour cream, or total substitution of yogurt for sour cream. Our families and friends seem to prefer yogurt as a topping for baked potatoes, and so might you.

We have left butter and margarine off the breads. You won't miss them when the bread has high quality and good flavor. To make dressing we use a mix of half extra-virgin olive oil (with its wonderful flavor) and half balsamic vinegar (a sweet, flavorful aged wine vinegar).

Portion sizes fit the food-pyramid guidelines. Most meat or cheese servings are no more than four ounces. We encourage you to fill up on fresh fruit, vegetables, bread, pasta, and rice. Although we prefer to cook our own beans, we suggest canned beans here for convenience, even though that adds a bit more sodium than we prefer.

Enjoy!

Dingers

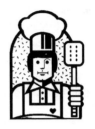

Menus

Salmon Steaks with *Pommery-Mustard Sauce* alongside
New Potatoes and *Vegetables*

Fresh Shrimp served with *Saffron Rice* and *Brussels Sprouts*

Black Bean Soup served with *French Bread* and *Romaine Salad with Arugula*

Cornish Game Hen served over *Wild Rice Bounty* with *Asparagus Spears*

Beef Tenderloin served alongside *Tomato Concassé* and *Baked Potato with Yogurt Cream*

Ginger Chicken served over *Jasmine Rice* with *Broccoli* and *Tomatoes*

Filipino Stir-Fry over Noodles

Lunches

Broiled Herbed Turkey Fajitas with banana slices

Tropical Fruit Salad with *Crusty French Bread and Cheese* and low-fat yogurt

Sweet Lentil Soup, hard rolls, and apple slices

Smoked Salmon and Fresh Dill on rye with ripe red grapes

Vegetable Carousel and Pasta Salad with fresh orange slices

Tomato-Basil Pita with carrot sticks

Spinach Salad with Gorgonzola Cheese and whole-grain bread

Breakfasts

Apricot-Fig Granola

Banana-Raisin Granola

Zucchini-Fig Muffins with *Fruit Kabobs*

Almond-Peach Muffins

French Toast with cantaloupe wedge

Pineapple-Banana Bread and low-fat yogurt

Apple Blueberry Crisp

Salmon Steaks with Pommery-Mustard Sauce alongside New Potatoes and Vegetables

Salmon Steaks (4 servings)

Salmon steaks	16 oz.(4–4 oz. steaks)
Lemon juice	2 Tbsp.
Black pepper	1 tsp.
Vegetable cooking spray	as needed

Preheat oven to 400° F. Lightly spray aluminum foil with cooking spray. Arrange steaks in single layer. Sprinkle juice lightly over steaks. Grind fresh pepper over steaks. Fold foil over steaks and seal well; place on baking sheet. Bake about 15 minutes.

Note: This is a simple, fail-safe way to prepare salmon, but you can grill or broil the salmon and serve the sauce on the side.

Pommery-Mustard Sauce (4 servings)

Fish stock or clam juice	6 oz.
Shallots	2 Tbsp.
Pommery mustard	4 tsp.
Tomatoes, diced	4 tsp.
Fresh chives	4 tsp.

Heat fish stock or clam juice and shallots in sauce pan over moderately high heat until volume is reduced by half. Mix in mustard and remove from heat. Add diced tomatoes and chives.

New Potatoes   *(4 servings)*

New potatoes (small)	16
Water	1/4 cup
Fresh parsley, finely chopped	1/3 cup

Scrub potatoes and rinse well with water. Steam until barely soft (8-10 mins.). Toss with parsley.

Vegetables   *(4 servings)*

Baby carrots	1/2 cup
Cherry tomatoes, halved	1/2 cup
Snow peas, stringy ends removed	1/2 cup
Baby yellow squash	1/2 cup
Water	2 Tbsp.

Rinse all vegetables. Add carrots to microwave-safe dish with the water. Cover the dish loosely. Microwave on high for two minutes. Add the remaining vegetables and microwave until all vegetables are just tender

Place salmon in center of dinner plate. Cover with sauce. Arrange vegetables and potatoes around it.

Dinners

Shrimp   _(4 servings)_

Olive oil	2 tsp.
Garlic, minced	2 cloves
Shrimp, peeled and deveined	16 medium

Fresh Shrimp served with Saffron Rice and _Brussels Sprouts_

In a heavy non-stick skillet, heat the oil until hot. Sauté the garlic until lightly browned. Add the shrimp and stir-fry for 1 min. or until the shrimp are opaque. Remove from heat.

Saffron Rice   _(4 servings)_

Rice, brown	2/3 cup
Stock (chicken or fish) or water	1 2/3 cup
Saffron	1/4 tsp.

Bring stock (fat skimmed, unsalted) or water to a boil in a medium saucepan and add rice. Return to boil and then turn heat down to simmer. Add saffron and stir. Cover. Simmer 60 mins. or until the water is absorbed.

Brussels Sprouts   _(4 servings)_

Brussels sprouts	16-20
Water	1/8 cup

Rinse sprouts and cut off stems. Place in dish. Add water, cover, and microwave until just tender.

Serve shrimp over rice, alongside Brussels sprouts.

Black Bean Soup   *(4 servings)*

Onion, small, chopped	1
Celery stalk, chopped	1
Carrot, chopped	1
Green pepper, finely chopped	1
Garlic, minced	2 cloves
Cumin, ground	1 tsp.
Black beans, canned	2 16-oz. cans
Chicken stock, defatted, reduced-sodium	2 cups
Dry sherry	2 tsp.
Fresh cilantro, finely chopped	4 Tbsp.

Combine onion, celery, carrot, and pepper in a microwave-safe dish. Add 2 Tbsp. water. Cover. Microwave on high until just tender. Transfer to a blender or food processor. Add garlic, cumin, and one can beans. Purée until smooth. Transfer to a Dutch oven. Add chicken stock. Drain and rinse the remaining beans and add to pot. Heat soup to piping hot. Stir in sherry and cilantro one or two minutes before serving.

Black Bean Soup* served with French bread and *Tangy Salad

Tangy Salad   *(4 servings)*

Balsamic vinegar	1 Tbsp.
Olive oil, extra virgin	1 Tbsp.
Romaine lettuce	3 cups
Arugula	1 cup
Red onion, sliced thinly	1/4 cup
Tomato, sliced	1/2 cup

Mix vinegar and oil. Set aside. Wash and tear the lettuce leaves. Wash and tear arugula leaves. Toss all the vegetables with vinegar and oil.

Serve the soup and salad together, with a nice, crusty French bread. Heating the bread in an oven on a cookie sheet will increase its crustiness and flavor.

Cornish Game Hen   *(4 servings)*

Cornish Game Hen served over **Wild Rice Bounty** with **Asparagus Spears**

Cornish game hen	1
Onion, coarsely chopped	1 small
Garlic, finely chopped	1 clove
Lemon, quartered	1/2

Combine onion, lemon, and garlic. Lightly place in hen (do not pack). Bake hen in oven dish at 325° F for 1 hour. Discard seasonings.

Save drippings for *Wild Rice Bounty*.

Wild Rice Bounty   *(4 servings)*

Water	4 cups
Wild rice	1 cup
Scallions, chopped fine	4
Mushrooms, sliced	8 oz. fresh or 6 oz. canned
Drippings from game hen, skimmed of fat	
White pepper	to taste
Salt	1/4 tsp.

In a medium saucepan, bring water to a boil and add rice and salt. Simmer, covered for 60 mins. or until rice absorbs all the water. Lightly sauté scallions and mushrooms in a non-stick skillet in drippings and season with white pepper. As soon as the rice is done, add the other ingredients. Mix and cover. Stir occasionally to avoid stickiness while holding for service.

Asparagus Spears   *(4 servings)*

Asparagus spears	16–20
Lemon slices	8

Trim and peel asparagus, peeling from butt end toward tip. Place in a microwave-safe dish with ends pointing outward. Add water and cover loosely. Microwave on high until just tender and bright green. Serve with fresh lemon slices.

Mound *Wild Rice Bounty* beside the hen, and fan the spears alongside.

Beef Tenderloin
(4 servings)

Beef tenderloin	4 4-oz.
Black pepper, freshly ground	1 tsp.
Vegetable cooking spray	as needed
Soy sauce, reduced sodium	1 Tbsp.

Preheat oven to broil. Season meat with pepper. Broil for 8–10 mins on lightly sprayed baking sheet, basting with soy sauce.

Beef Tenderloin served alongside Tomato Concassé and Baked Potato with Yogurt Sour Cream

Baked Potato with Yogurt Cream
(4 servings)

Potato, white baking or russet	4
Yogurt, plain lowfat	4 Tbsp.
Sour cream	4 Tbsp.
Chives	4 Tbsp.

Scrub potatoes and pierce skin several times. Bake at 425° F until potatoes are tender, about 45 mins. Mix yogurt, sour cream, and chives. Split potatoes immediately. Add yogurt mix.

Tomato Concassé
(4 servings)

Ripe plum tomatoes	8
Olive oil	1 tsp.
Shallots, minced	2 Tbsp.
Garlic, crushed and chopped	1 clove
Fresh oregano	1 tsp.

Peel and dice tomatoes.* Chop oregano and garlic. Heat oil gently in sauce pan, add garlic and shallots, and cook until lightly browned. Add tomatoes and oregano and cook for 2 mins. Remove from heat. Serve with meat.

*Buy already peeled, canned plum tomatoes or dip fresh tomatoes in boiling water for 30 sec. and peel.

Serve the beef tenderloin alongside the tomato concassé and potato.

Ginger Chicken
(4 servings)

Ginger Chicken served over *Jasmine Rice* with *Broccoli* and *Tomatoes*

Chicken breast, boneless and skinless	2

Marinade:

Soy sauce, reduced sodium	4 Tbsp.
White wine	1/4 cup
Lemon juice	2 Tbsp.
Ginger, peeled, grated	3 Tbsp.
Garlic, minced	1 clove
Crushed red pepper	1/4 tsp.
Dijon mustard	1 tsp.

Wash and trim chicken of any excess fat. Slice into bite-size pieces. In a blender or food processor, combine marinade ingredients and blend well. Add marinade to chicken and marinate for at least 1 hour or overnight. Heat a skillet over medium heat. Cook chicken in marinade. Stir frequently.

Jasmine Rice

Jasmine rice*	1 cup
Water	1 3/4 cups

Wash rice with cold water. In a small saucepan, bring water to a boil. Add rice, cover, and simmer for 15 mins. or until water is absorbed. (If using rice cooker, follow those instructions.)

*Jasmine rice is available in most grocery stores with a well-stocked Oriental food section.

Broccoli and Tomatoes
(4 servings)

Broccoli	1 1/2 cup
Water	1/8 cup
Tomatoes, diced	1 cup

Wash broccoli. Cut into small flowerets. Place broccoli, ends pointing outward, and water into microwave-safe dish. Cover loosely and microwave until just tender. Mix broccoli and tomatoes with Ginger Chicken and serve over a bed of jasmine rice.

Filipino Stir Fry over Noodles   *(4 servings)*

Japanese noodles or Angel hair pasta	12 oz.
Water	3 cups
Chicken breast, boneless and skinless	1 large breast or 2 halves
Olive oil	2 tsp.
Garlic, minced	1 clove
Black pepper, freshly ground	1 tsp.
Carrots, diagonally sliced	1 cup
Napa cabbage, roughly chopped	1/8 head
Snow peas	1 cup
Soy sauce, reduced sodium	2 Tbsp.
Lemon juice	4 Tbsp.
Scallions, chopped	3 Tbsp.

***Filipino Stir-Fry* served over noodles (or angel-hair pasta)**

Boil water and pour over Japanese noodles. Let soak until tender. Set aside. (Drain before using.) If using angel hair pasta, bring water to boil, cut noodles in half, and cook for 10-15 mins. Drain. Wash and slice chicken into bite-size pieces. Heat oil in large skillet or wok. Add garlic and heat until lightly browned. Add chicken and cook while stirring frequently. Spread scallions over top of noodles. Season chicken with pepper, lemon juice, and soy sauce. Add carrots and cook 1-2 mins. Add cabbage and snow peas, stirring frequently. Place stir fry on warmed noodles.

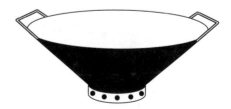

___

Broiled
Herbed Turkey
Fajitas with
sliced bananas

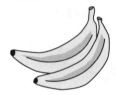

Broiled Herbed Turkey Fajitas   *(4 servings)*

Garlic, minced	2 cloves
Fresh herbs: rosemary, thyme, & oregano	1 Tbsp. each
Lemon juice	2 Tbsp.
Olive oil	2 tsp.
Vegetable cooking spray	As needed
Black pepper, freshly ground	1 tsp.
Turkey breasts, boneless and skinless	4 4-oz.
Red onions, thinly sliced	1/2 cup
Romaine lettuce	2 cups
Tomato, sliced	2 cups
Tortillas, steamed or lightly baked	4

Combine garlic, herbs, lemon juice, oil, and pepper. Mix well. Marinate turkey in mixture for at least 10 mins. Longer is better. Set oven to broil. Spray a baking tray, set turkey on it. Broil turkey strips on one side for 3–4 mins. Turn and broil for 3–4 mins. more. Put lettuce on the warm tortilla, add turkey, onions, and tomatoes, and fold up tortilla.

Serve with four sliced bananas.

Tropical Fruit Salad   *(4 servings)*

Tropical Fruit
Salad with
Crusty French
Bread and
Cheese

Apple	1
Kiwi	3
Mango	2
Orange	1
Banana	2
Papaya	1
Orange juice	1/2 cup

Peel and slice all the fruit and mix with orange juice.

Serve with Crusty French Bread and Cheese (at right).

Crusty French Bread and Cheese   *(4 servings)*

French bread, crusty baguette	4–6 slices
Cheese, brie or camembert (room temperature)	2 oz.

Slice bread and spread with cheeses.

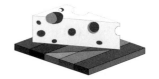

Sweet Lentil Soup   *(4 servings)*

Chicken broth, low-sodium	4 cups
Lentils, brown	1/2 cup
Carrots, obliquely chopped	1 cup
Celery, chopped	1 cup
Potato, cubed	1 small
Onion, chopped	1 medium
Lentils, red	1/2 cup
Mango chutney	2 Tbsp.
Black pepper, freshly ground	1 tsp.

Sweet Lentil Soup and hard rolls with apple slices

Rinse both batches of lentils separately. Combine broth, brown lentils, carrots, celery, potato, and onion. Bring to a boil and reduce heat. Add red lentils, cover, and simmer for 35 mins. Stir in mango chutney five minutes before removing from heat. Season with pepper.

Serve with four hard rolls and four sliced apples, such as McIntosh, Ida Red, or Golden Delicious.

Smoked Salmon with Fresh Dill

    (4 servings)

Smoked salmon, thinly sliced	4 oz.
Rye bread	4–8 slices
Fresh dill	2–4 Tbs.

Smoked Salmon and Fresh Dill on rye with ripe red grapes

Place salmon on slices of rye bread and liberally cover with fresh dill.

Serve with 1 pound of grapes.

Vegetable Carousel and Pasta Salad   *(4 servings)*

***Vegetable Carousel and Pasta Salad* with fresh orange slices**

Water	2 cups
Bowtie pasta	1 cup
Red pepper	1
Yellow squash, lightly steamed	1/2 medium
Cucumber, chopped and quartered	1/4 cup
Red onion, thinly sliced	1/4 cup
Balsamic vinegar	1 Tbsp.
Olive oil	1 Tbsp.
Sugar	1 tsp.
Parsley, coarsely chopped	2 Tbsp.

Bring water to a boil and cook pasta. Meanwhile, wash all vegetables. Julienne cut peppers and squash.* Cut other vegetables. Mix vinegar, oil and sugar. When pasta is done, drain and toss with parsley, vegetables, and vinegar-oil mixture.

*A julienne cut makes rectangular pieces 2–3" long. Trim the vegetable so that the sides are straight. Slice lengthwise. Stack the slices and cut into strips.

Slice four oranges. A peeled orange with white membrane removed and sliced into "wheels" makes a nice presentation to accompany the pasta.

Tomato-Basil Pita *(4 servings)*

Pitas	4
Plum tomato, chopped	4
Basil, fresh chopped	2 Tbsp.
Balsamic vinegar	2 tsp.
Cucumber	1/2 cup
Alfalfa sprouts	1/2 cup
Romaine lettuce leaves	8

Combine tomatoes, basil, and vinegar. Add cucumbers and alfalfa. Wash and dry lettuce and line pita. Fill with tomatoes, basil, cucumbers, and alfalfa sprouts.

Cut 4–6 carrots into sticks and serve as an accompaniment.

Tomato-Basil Pita with carrot sticks

Spinach Salad with Gorgonzola Cheese
(4 servings)

Spinach leaves	4 cups
Carrots, julienned	1/2 cup
Red onions, thinly sliced	1/2 onion
Vinaigrette*	2 tsp.
Gorgonzola cheese	2 oz.
Eggs, hard-boiled, chopped	1

Wash spinach thoroughly. Tear clean spinach leaves into bowl. Add vegetables and vinaigrette and toss well. Crumble Gorgonzola over salad. Top with eggs.

Vinaigrette:

Olive oil	1/2 cup
Balsamic vinegar	1/2 cup
Basil, chopped or dried	2 tsp.

Serve the salad with 4 to 8 slices of whole-grain bread, fresh fruit or low-fat fruited yogurt.

Spinach Salad with Gorgonzola Cheese and whole-grain bread

Breakfasts

Apricot-Fig Granola

or

Banana-Raisin Granola

Apricot-Fig Granola *(4 servings)*

Rolled oats	1/2 cup
Rolled wheat or wheat bran	1/2 cup
Grape Nuts	1 cup
Figs, dried, chopped	8
Apricots, dried, chopped	8
Almonds	1/4 cup

Mix all ingredients.

Banana-Raisin Granola *(4 servings)*

Rolled oats	1/2 cup
Oat bran	1/2 cup
Wheat germ	1/2 cup
Raisins	1/4 cup
Dried prunes	8
Sunflower seeds	2 Tbs.

Mix all ingredients. Add sliced banana just before serving.

Serve granola with skim milk.

Zucchini-Fig Muffins   *(12 muffins)*

Vegetable oil	3 Tbsp.
Vanilla extract	2 tsp.
Egg whites	3
Honey	2 Tbsp.
Sugar	1 cup
Cinnamon	2 tsp.
Wheat bran	2/3 cup
Zucchini, grated	1 medium
Flour, all-purpose	1 cup
Flour, whole-wheat	1 cup
Dried figs, chopped	1 cup
Baking soda	1 tsp.
Baking powder	1 tsp.

Zucchini-Fig Muffins with Fruit Kabobs

Preheat oven to 425° F. Coat muffin tin with vegetable cooking spray. In large bowl, blend oil, vanilla, egg whites, honey, sugar, cinnamon. Stir in wheat bran, zucchini, and raisins. In another large bowl, sift together flour, baking soda, and baking powder. Mix in wet ingredients until flour mixture is just moistened. Spoon into muffin cups until 3/4 full. Bake on middle oven rack for 15–18 mins. or until browned. Let cool on rack. Note: Muffins can be frozen.

Fruit Kabobs   *(4 servings)*

Strawberries, halved	4
Kiwi	1
Mango	1
Pineapple	1/2 cup
Honeydew	1/4 melon

Wash and cut all fruit into bite-size pieces. Assemble on 4 12-inch skewers and serve with muffins

Note: Slice the mango twice, once alongside each side of the seed. Slice diamond pattern in each half and scoop out fruit.

Almond-Peach Muffins *(12 muffins)*

Almond-Peach Muffins

Skim milk	1 cup
Peach, peeled, chopped	2
Sugar	1/2 cup
Vegetable oil	2 Tbsp.
Egg white	1 large
Almond extract	2 Tbsp.
Flour, all-purpose	1 cup
Flour, whole-wheat	1 cup
Rolled oats	1/2 cup
Baking soda	1 tsp.
Baking powder	1 tsp.
Almonds, sliced	1/4 cup

Preheat oven to 425° F. Lightly oil muffin tin. In blender, combine: milk, 1 peach, sugar, oil, egg white, and extract. Stir in remaining chopped peach. In large bowl, sift together: flour, baking soda, and baking powder. Stir in oats. Make a hole in the mound of flour and pour in peach mixture. Mix until flour mixture is just moistened. Spoon into muffin tins. Top with almonds. Bake on middle oven rack for 15–18 mins. or until lightly browned. Let cool on rack. *Note:* Muffins can be frozen.

Enjoy with orange juice or skim milk.

French Toast with a canteloupe wedge

French Toast *(4 servings)*

Egg	2
Egg white	2
Cinnamon	2 tsp.
Allspice	1/2 tsp.
Sugar	2 tsp.
Whole-grain bread	8 slices
Maple syrup	8 Tbsp.

Beat together eggs, egg whites, cinnamon, allspice, and sugar. Dip both sides of bread into egg mixture. Cook on nonstick skillet, 2–3 mins. on each side. Serve with maple syrup.

Serve with a cantaloupe wedge.

Pineapple-Banana Bread (12 servings)

Vegetable oil	1 tsp.
Sugar	2/3 cup
Banana, mashed	1 cup
Pineapple, crushed	1/2 cup
Flour, all-purpose	1 3/4 cup
Baking soda	1/2 tsp.
Baking powder	2 tsp.
Eggs	2
Nuts, chopped	1/4 cup

Pineapple-Banana Bread and low-fat yogurt

Preheat oven to 350° F. Coat loaf pan with vegetable cooking spray. In a blender or food processor combine sugar, banana, pineapple, and oil. In a large bowl, sift together flour, baking soda, and baking powder. Make a well in the flour mound and pour in half wet mixture. Add beaten eggs. Stir. Add remaining wet mixture and nuts and stir until just moistened. Bake for 55-60 mins. Let cool in pan for 5 mins. and then transfer to a cooling rack.

Apple-Blueberry Crisp (4 servings)

Cornstarch	1 tsp.
Blueberries	3/4 lb.
Granny Smith apples	1 cup
Cinnamon	1 tsp.
Flour	1 1/2 Tbsp.
Sugar	1/4 cup
Rolled oats	3/4 cup
Grape Nuts or wheat germ	1/4 cup

Blend 1/4 lb. of blueberries and cornstarch. Toss whole blueberries, apples, sugar, flour, and cinnamon with half of blended blueberry mixture. Place in a non-stick baking dish. Combine oats, Grape Nuts, and remaining blueberry mixture until moistened. Sprinkle over apple-blueberry mixture and bake at 350° F for 40 mins. or until hot and bubbly.

Enjoy warm crisp with a glass of skim milk, or top with low-fat yogurt.

Glossary

Aerobic exercise—Exercise that promotes oxygen use in your body.

Achilles' tendon—A thick cord in the back of the ankle that controls much of the foot's movement.

Adrenaline—A body chemical that energizes and strengthens the system for immediate action.

Anaerobic exercise—Physical exertion that does not promote the use of oxygen by the body, usually characterized by short bursts of activity.

Anthropometric measurements—Measuring the human body.

Autonomous exercisers—People for whom exercise has become part of their routine.

Autonomy—Making one's own decisions and controlling one's activities.

Body-composition analysis—An assessment of the relative amounts of lean and fat tissue.

Beta-carotene—A nutrient associated with orange-colored vegetables that is converted into vitamin A in the body.

Calisthenics—Light exercises, usually repetitive, such as sit-ups and jumping jacks.

Carotid artery—The vessel that supplies blood to the head and is easily found in the neck to count pulse rate.

Cardiovascular system—Lungs, heart, and blood vessels.

Cholesterol—A waxy substance needed for proper body functions, but dangerous if it sticks to and clogs arteries.

Degenerative diseases—Conditions in which body functions are gradually impaired or lost, such as osteoporosis (thinning bones) and heart disease.

Dehydration—Loss of water in the body.

Depression—Low spirits or low vitality.

Detoxifying diet—A false theory of nutrition based on misinformation.

Duration—The length of time exercising at the target heart rate.

Endorphins—Body chemicals that produce soothing effects.

Endurance—Capacity for prolonged activity.

Extensor mechanism—Muscles that move arms or legs away from the body.

Fat-soluble vitamins—Micronutrients that are stored in the body's fat cells until needed (e.g., vitamins A, D, and K).

Flexometer—A measuring device for muscle flexibility.

Food groups—Groupings of related foods, for the purpose of assembling a balanced diet.

Food pyramid—A way of picturing the recommendation that people obtain the bulk of their calories from breads, grains, fruits, and vegetables (the base of the pyramid), while limiting meats, dairy, and fat (the top of the pyramid).

Frequency—The number of exercise sets in a week.

Geriatric research—Studies of aged people.

Hierarchy of human needs—A widely accepted theory that people who satisfy certain basic needs, such as food and safety, will then seek higher-level needs, such as love and esteem.

Hypotheses—Assumptions or ideas to be tested.

Hydration—Volume of water in the body.

Intensity—The level of effort used to perform an activity.

Intrinsic—Inside or within.

Isometric training—Exercises involving pushing against or pulling unmoving objects.

Isotonic training—Exercises involving lifting a load to move a muscle through its full range of motion.

Isokinetic lifting—Exercises that move muscles in specific ways using specialized equipment.

Ligament—Connective tissue that joins bones in joints.

Lipids—Fats.

Metabolism—The chemical processes in a person's cells, particularly the generation of energy.

Monounsaturated fat—With a variant chemical formula, thought to be the fat least harmful to humans.

Morbidity—Disease.

Muscle tone—Condition of muscles; good muscle tone implies firm muscles.

Neurobiology—The study of the nervous system.

Nutrient density—The relationship of the amount of nutrition in a food to the calories supplied by that food. Foods nearest their natural state have the highest nutrient density.

Obesity—A level of excess fat tissue that threatens health.

Opposing muscles—Muscles working in pairs opposite each other. Usually one extends and the other retracts.

Polyunsaturated fats—A form of fat thought to have fewer links to heart disease than saturated fat.

Psychoneuroimmunology—The concept that the mind has considerable control over a person's physical health.

Psychopharmacological drugs—Chemicals that alter a person's mood or consciousness.

Radial artery—The vessel that supplies blood to the hand and is easily found in the wrist to count pulse rate.

Range of motion—The distance within the limits of a muscle's ability to move.

RDI (recommended daily intake)—A term instituted in 1994 for target amounts for each day's consumption of food nutrients, replacing USRDA.

RDV (recommended daily values)—Similar to RDV, another term for target amounts for each day's consumption of food nutrients, replacing USRDA.

Repetitions—Repeated controlled movements to exercise a particular muscle or group of muscles.

Respiration—The use of oxygen by body cells to create energy.

Saturated fat—A substance linked to heart disease.

Sedentary—Accustomed to sitting or inactivity.

Self-esteem—A favorable opinion of oneself, but not at the expense of others.

Self love—Taking care of oneself physically and mentally to allow one to give more service to the world, not to be confused with selfishness.

Serving size—One unit of a given food, used as a means to count the relative amounts of different food groups consumed in a day.

Set point—The theoretical "proper" weight established by a person's genetic and environmental influences. Efforts to gain or lose weight beyond the set point are often unsuccessful.

Sit-and-reach test—A means of measuring flexibility by having a person stretch forward while sitting flat on the floor.

Skinfold-caliper technique—A means of assessing amounts of lean and fat tissue by gently squeezing and measuring a portion of skin and associated flesh.

Statistical significance—A mathematical calculation of certainty, usually expressed as a p value, that a given study result did not occur merely by chance. A p less than .05 indicates no more than a 5-percent probability that a mathematical result occurred by chance.

Stroke—An interruption of blood to the brain that often causes lasting damage and loss of function.

Supplements —Vitamin and mineral pills that purport to improve on a good diet or make up for a poor one.

Target heart rate—A heartbeat pace that is appropriate or desirable during exercise.

Type-A behavior—A lifestyle of high pressure and quick action often thought to be connected to heart attacks.

USRDA (United States recommended daily allowance)—The term used starting in 1978 for recommendations from government agencies regarding target amounts for each day's consumption of food nutrients.

Water-soluble vitamins—Micronutrients that are not stored in the body but are excreted when in excess (e.g., vitamins B and C).

Wellness—Having a healthy, well-adjusted lifestyle, with positive physical and mental frames of reference.

Index